Current Communications

GY

1988

ts

Titles in
Current Communications in Molecular Biology
PLANT INFECTIOUS AGENTS
ENHANCERS AND EUKARYOTIC GENE EXPRESSION
PROTEIN TRANSPORT AND SECRETION
IMMUNE RECOGNITION OF PROTEIN ANTIGENS
EUKARYOTIC TRANSCRIPTION
PLANT CELL/CELL INTERACTIONS
TRANSLATIONAL CONTROL
COMPUTER GRAPHICS AND MOLECULAR MODELING
MICROBIAL ENERGY TRANSDUCTION
MECHANISMS OF YEAST RECOMBINATION
DNA PROBES
ANGIOGENESIS: Mechanisms and Pathobiology
GENE TRANSFER VECTORS FOR MAMMALIAN CELLS
INOSITOL LIPIDS IN CELLULAR SIGNALING
NUCLEAR ONCOGENES
GENETIC IMPROVEMENTS OF AGRICULTURALLY IMPORTANT CROPS: Progress and Issues

GENETIC IMPROVEMENTS OF AGRICULTURALLY IMPORTANT CROPS: Progress and Issues
Copyright 1988 by Cold Spring Harbor Laboratory
All rights reserved
International Standard Book Number 0-87969-305-3
Book design by Emily Harste
Printed in the United States of America

Cover: Photo courtesy of Curt Maas, Pioneer Hi-Bred International, Inc.

All Cold Spring Harbor Laboratory publications may be ordered directly from Cold Spring Harbor Laboratory, Box 100, Cold Spring Harbor, New York 11724. (Phone: Continental U.S. except New York State 1-800-843-4388. All other locations [516] 367-8325.)

Conference Participants

Susan B. Altenbach, The Plant Cell Research Institute, Inc., Dublin, California

Charles J. Arntzen, du Pont Experimental Station, Wilmington, Delaware

Roger N. Beachy, Department of Biology, Washington University, St. Louis, Missouri

John Bedbrook, Advanced Genetic Sciences, Oakland, California

Philip Dale, IPSR Cambridge Laboratory, England

Nina Fedoroff, Department of Embryology, Carnegie Institution of Washington, Baltimore, Maryland

Robert T. Fraley, Plant Molecular Biology Group, Monsanto Company, St. Louis, Missouri

Nicholas M. Frey, Department of Biotechnology, Pioneer Hi-Bred International, Inc., Johnston, Iowa

Tim Helentjaris, Molecular Biology Group, Native Plants, Inc., Salt Lake City, Utah

Robert B. Horsch, Department of Crop Transformation, Monsanto Company, St. Louis, Missouri

Christopher J. Lamb, Department of Plant Biology, The Salk Institute, San Diego, California

Jan J. Leemans, Plant Genetic Systems, Gent, Belgium

Catherine J. Mackey, Pfizer Central Research, Groton, Connecticut

James H. Maryanski, U.S. Food and Drug Administration, Washington, D.C.

Phyllis B. Moses, Board on Agriculture, National Research Council, Washington, D.C.

J. Brian Mudd, The Plant Cell Research Institute, Inc., Dublin, California

Steven Poe, U.S. Department of Agriculture, Hyattsville, Maryland

Patricia Roberts, U.S. Environmental Protection Agency, Washington, D.C.

Stephen Rothstein, Ciba-Geigy Corporation, Research Triangle Park, North Carolina

Vernon W. Ruttan, Department of Applied and Agricultural Economics, University of Minnesota, St. Paul

Jeff Schell, Max-Planck-Institut für Zuchtungsforschung, Koln, Federal Republic of Germany

Michael M. Simpson, Life Sciences Section, Congressional Research Service, Washington, D.C.

Jerry L. Slighton, Department of Molecular Biology, The Upjohn Company, Kalamazoo, Michigan

David M. Stalker, Calgene Inc., Davis, California

Arthur Weissinger, Pioneer Hi-Bred International, Inc., Johnston, Iowa

The meeting on Genetic Improvements of Agriculturally Important Crops was funded entirely by proceeds from the Laboratory's Corporate Sponsor Program, whose members provide core support for Cold Spring Harbor and Banbury meetings:

Abbot Laboratories
American Cyanamid Company
Amersham International plc
AMGen
Becton Dickinson and Company
Boehringer Mannheim GmbH
Bristol-Myers Company
Cetus Corporation
Ciba-Geigy Corporation
Diagnostic Products Corporation
E.I. du Pont de Nemours & Company
Eastman Kodak Company
Genentech, Inc.
Genetics Institute
Hoffmann-La Roche Inc.
Johnson & Johnson
Eli Lilly and Company
Millipore Corporation
Monsanto Company
Oncogene Science, Inc.
Pall Corporation
Pfizer Inc.
The Procter & Gamble Company
Schering-Plough Corporation
Smith Kline & French Laboratories
Tambrands Inc.
The Upjohn Company
The Wellcome Research Laboratories,
  Burroughs Wellcome Co.
Wyeth Laboratories

Preface

Improvements in agricultural productivity rely in part on the creation procedures of new varieties through breeding. Recently, the scope of scientific tools that can be brought to bear on plant breeding has been dramatically broadened by the introduction of tissue-culture techniques based on advancing knowledge of plant cellular biology and of genetic engineering techniques based on knowledge about plant gene structure and function.

Progress has been very rapid, and an increasing number of new varieties obtained by a combination of these methods must now be tested in the field. It was therefore time to bring together various academic and industrial researchers and officials from the government agencies (USDA, EPA, and FDA). The aim of this meeting was to assess the scientific and technical progress and to ponder the impact of this progress on agriculture. A particular focus was a candid discussion of the regulatory process controlling the release of new crop varieties. Such a regulatory process should satisfy both legitimate concerns regarding environmental impact and health and the need to let research and development proceed in a rational and efficient way.

It was the late Steve Prentis who had realized the need and timeliness of such a discussion and offered to organize it in the exceptionally appropriate surroundings of the Banbury Center. The quality and intensity of the intellectual exchanges have shown that Steve Prentis had been right. The organization was up to its best standards thanks to Terri Grodzicker and Bea Toliver of the Banbury Center. All the participants will carry very fond memories of the warm hospitality provided in Robertson House by Katya Davey and her staff. Sincere thanks are also due to Nancy Ford, Nadine Dumser, and Mary Cozza for their outstanding work in editing and publishing this book.

N.M.F
R.T.F
J.S.

Contents

Introduction

N.M. Frey

Plant Breeding Division, Pioneer Hi-Bred International
Johnston, Illinois 50131

Until 1982, genetic improvement of agriculturally important crops relied solely either on sexual recombination followed by selection or, to a lesser degree, on random or induced mutations. In 1982, direct gene transfers became possible using recombinant DNA technologies (DeBlock et al. 1984; Horsch et al. 1984). This plant breeding approach has resulted in genetic improvements in productivity of 0.5% to more than 1.0% per year for the major agronomic crops, including maize, soybean, and wheat (Fehr 1984). The discovery of molecular techniques to transfer genes among organisms without sexual crossing provides geneticists new opportunities to improve the efficiency of production and to increase the utility of our agricultural crops. Plants with new traits such as herbicide resistance, insect resistance, virus resistance, and fungal resistance have been developed using genes from unrelated organisms. Researchers are also trying to enhance the utility of our agricultural produce by altering the nutritional quality of proteins and oils.[1]

These new opportunities to augment the genetic improvements that plant breeders continue to make in our agricultural crops have raised questions about how safe our future agricultural produce will be for consumption. The products of plant breeding have not historically required regulatory approval before commercial sale. Plant products developed using recombinant DNA technology, however, now require regulatory approval before initial field testing can be conducted. Although a National Academy of Sciences' paper (Kelman et al. 1987) concluded that, "The risks associated with the introduction of recombinant-DNA-engineered organisms are the same in kind as those associated with the introduction into the environment of unmodified organisms or organisms modified by other genetic techniques," a Coordinated Framework for Regulation of

---

[1]The papers published in this book provide referenced examples for the reader.

Biotechnology (Office of Science and Technology Policy 1986) has been developed to provide regulatory oversight for the products of recombinant DNA research.

The development of recombinant DNA technology has moved molecular biologists, plant breeders, and government regulators into uncharted territory. The science is developing, potential new plant products are being identified, and new regulations are being developed. The purpose of this meeting was to bring together people representing each of these areas—science, product development, and government—to establish a dialog focused on the issues important to the development of this new technology for the benefit of agriculture and the consuming public.

REFERENCES

DeBlock, M., L. Herrera-Estrella, M. van Montagu, J. Schell, and P. Zambryski. 1984. Expression of foreign genes in regenerated plants and their progeny. *EMBO J.* **3(8):** 1681.

Fehr, W.R. 1984. Genetic contributions to yield gains of five major crop plants. In *CSSA Special Publication No. 7.* Crop Science Society of America, Madison, Wisconsin.

Horsch, R.B., R.T. Fraley, S.G. Rogers, P.R. Sanders, A. Lloyd, and N. Hoffmann. 1984. Inheritance of functional foreign genes in plants. *Science* **223:** 496.

Kelman, A., W. Anderson, S. Faklow, N.V. Fedoroff, and S. Levin. 1987. Introduction of recombinant DNA-engineered organisms into the environment: Key issues. Prepared for the Council of the National Academy of Sciences, Washington, D.C.

Office of Science and Technology Policy. 1986. Part II. Coordinated framework for regulation of biotechnology. *Federal Register* **51(123):** 23302.

Plant Transformation Using *Agrobacterium* and Direct DNA Uptake Methods

J. Schell

Max-Planck-Institut für Züchtungsforschung, 5000 Cologne 30
Federal Republic of Germany

Gene-vector systems based on the natural capacity of *Agrobacterium* strains to transfer and integrate DNA segments in the plant genome have been improved, diversified, and used to study the structure and function of regulatory DNA sequences specifying quantitative and qualitative gene expression. Improvements of gene-vector systems, based on the *Agrobacterium* Ti and Ri plasmids, offer a better understanding of the tDNA transfer mechanism.

Agrobacteria harboring the necessary virulence genes can transfer any DNA segment carried either on an extrachromosomal plasmid or on its chromosome, provided this DNA segment is bordered by a set of "integration sequences." These specific integration sequences are 25 bp in length and are recognized by the products of some of the Ti plasmid virulence genes (*virD*). Wounded plants release low-molecular-weight phenolic compounds that induce the virulence genes of agrobacteria, and the product of one of these virulence genes (*virD*) causes single-strand breaks in the 25-bp integration sequences. This, in turn, leads to the formation in the induced agrobacteria of a single-stranded copy (so-called T strand) of the DNA segment included between the repeated set of integration sequences (Wang et al. 1984; Stachel et al. 1985, 1986).

All of these observations are strikingly reminiscent of bacterial conjugation and led to the suggestion that tDNA transfer to plants might in fact be a (very) special type of conjugation, involving bacterial and plant cells (Wang et al. 1984; Stachel et al. 1986).

Indeed, single-stranded DNA intermediates involved in bacterial conjugation are initiated by the introduction of a specific nick at *oriT* by so-called *mob* functions (Everett and Willetts 1980). The question, therefore, was whether the *virD*-tDNA border sequence system would be the functional equivalent of the *mob-oriT* system of bacterial conjugation. This appears to be the case with regard to wide-host-range plasmid RSF1010 because this plasmid carrying a plant-selectable marker gene was shown to be transferred and integrated into plant cells (Buchanan-Wollaston et al. 1987). *vir* functions (other than *virD*), as well as *mob* and *oriT*, of RSF1010 were essential for this transfer to take place. It remains to be seen whether integration in plant DNA took place through the *oriT* sequence. These results also show that it is possible that a variety of wide-host-range plasmids can be transferred to plants via transition in agrobacteria and that, therefore, plants might have access to the gene pool of gram-negative bacteria.

It is not yet known how the single-stranded tDNA copy ultimately gets transferred to the plant cell and is integrated covalently as a double-stranded DNA insert at random sites in the nuclear plant DNA. However, the integration mechanism appears to be fairly precise because it involves sequences in or near the 25-bp integration sequences that flank the tDNA segment. Thus, any DNA sequence (up to 40 kb or more in length) that is flanked by the specific integration sequences and introduced into agrobacteria will be transferred by these bacteria to the plant cells (Zambryski et al. 1983; Bevan 1984; Fraley et al. 1985; Koncz and Schell 1986).

Special-purpose vectors for gene-expression studies, shotgun cloning, insertional mutagenesis in active genes, and the convenient regeneration of transformed cells into plants have been developed. Recent research is expanding the host range of such gene vectors to a large number of crop plants: tomato, potato, alfalfa, soya, brassica, sugar beet, and so forth. Promoter DNA sequences derived from tDNA genes or from plant viruses such as the cauliflower mosaic virus (and the wheat dwarf virus) were used successfully to express enzymes such as neomycin phosphotransferase (NPT), hygromycin phosphotransferasease (HPT), chloramphenicol acetyltransferase (CAT), methotrexate-resistant dehydrofolate reductase, enolpyruvate shikimate synthase, phosphinotrycine transacetylase, and others in plants.

Reporter Genes
To study the role of *cis*-active sequence elements in the regulation of gene expression, such sequences were combined with reporter-gene sequences. In most instances, *Escherichia coli* genes were used for this purpose. The most commonly used are

4

sequences coding for CAT or for the aminoglycoside phospho-transferase II from Tn5 (APHII). Both of these enzymes, particularly APHII, require relatively complex assay procedures, and the results are not easily quantified. Recently, two systems were developed to overcome these limitations: (1) Light-emitting luciferase enzymes were expressed in tobacco under the control of plant-specific expression sequences. In one instance, the luciferase-coding sequences were derived from the *luxA* and *luxB* cistrons of *Vibrio harveyi*. *luxA* and *luxB* "transcription-translation" cassettes were constructed and shown to be properly expressed in transgenic plants (Koncz et al. 1987a). The luciferase of fireflies was also shown to be functional in transgenic plants (Ow et al. 1986).

Recently, another very sensitive and highly promising reporter enzyme for work in plants was reported (Jefferson et al. 1987). The bacterial β-glucuronidase (GUS) is very stable in transgenic plants, and very easy and sensitive assays for this enzyme have been developed.

Study of *cis*-Active Sequence Elements Involved in Gene-expression Regulation

Light-regulated Gene Expression. Two types of genes have been studied extensively. The first type consists of nuclear genes such as the gene coding for the small subunit of the ribulose-1,5-bisphosphate carboxylase (*rbcS*) or the gene for the light-harvesting chlorophyll *a/b* protein (*LHCP*), whose products are active after transport into chloroplasts. These genes have been shown to be light inducible.

Phytochrome and, in the case of the *rbcS* gene, a blue light receptor were shown to convey the light signal needed for the expression of these genes. Finally, these genes were shown to be active only in tissues (such as green leaves) that contain active chloroplasts. Several studies involving individual *cab* and *rbcS* genes have shown that 5′ upstream sequences contained within the first few hundred base pairs upstream of the transcription initiation site of these genes are sufficient to confer light-inducible, phytochrome, and green chloroplast-dependent expression of a number of chimeric genes, expressing various reporter enzymes. The *cis*-acting sequences that are responsible for this regulated expression of chimeric genes were shown to be contained within small DNA sequences of no more than a few hundred base pairs. Some of these regulatory sequences were shown to work as light-dependent enhancers in leaves and as silencers in roots (Coruzzi et al. 1984; Herrera-Estrella et al. 1984; Morelli et al. 1985; Simpson et al. 1985, 1986; Timko et al. 1985; Tobin and Silverthorne 1985).

Chalcone synthase (CS) represents another type of light-regulated gene. Using 5′ upstream sequences from an *Antirrhinum majus* CS gene, it was possible to construct chimeric genes that would be silent in transgenic plants unless the plants were irradiated for 20 hours with ultraviolet (UV) light. Under continuous UV radiation for 20 hours, these transgenic plants transiently expressed the introduced chimeric genes at a high level (Kaulen et al. 1986).

Organ-specific Chimeric Genes. Sequences 5′ upstream derived from leaf-specific and tuber-specific genes have also been used to construct chimeric genes (Eckes et al. 1986; Rosahl et al. 1986 and in prep.). When such chimeric genes were introduced in transgenic plants, they were expressed with the same tight organ specificity as was the case for the original genes from which the 5′ upstream sequences were derived. It was also found that the patatin gene, which codes for a major reserve protein in potato tubers, could be made to produce stable patatin protein from a properly processed mRNA in the leaves of potato and tobacco transgenic plants simply by substituting its 5′ upstream sequences for those derived from a leaf-specific tobacco gene. These results therefore demonstrate that no organ-specific factors are involved in the splicing, processing, or translation of this tuber-specific gene.

Of particular interest are the observations made with the tuber-specific proteinase inhibitor II gene from potatoes. This gene is silent in potato leaves but is systemically induced throughout the plant as the result of the wounding of a single leaf or after treatment of detached leaves with oligosaccharides (Green and Ryan 1972; Ryan 1977; Keil et al. 1986; Sanchez-Serrano et al. 1986).

The tobacco genome does not carry genes homologous to the potato proteinase inhibitor II gene. When this gene was introduced in the tobacco genome (Sanchez-Serrano et al. 1987), no or very little expression was detected in nonwounded leaves, whereas high levels of proteinase inhibitor II mRNA were detected in leaves after mechanical wounding or after treatment with oligosaccharides. Wounding also led to a systemic induction in nonwounded leaves, stems, and roots. Obviously a hypothetical proteinase inhibitor-inducing factor (PIIF) must exist in tobacco for the induction of other genes and is also functional in inducing the potato gene.

Nodules can be considered as a special type of organ in legume species. Nodule-specific plant genes, called nodulins, have been identified and some, such as leghemoglobin, have been isolated (Bojsen et al. 1983; Lee et al. 1985). When a chimeric soybean leghemoglobin gene was introduced in the genome of another legume species, expression was found only in nodules and not in uninfected roots. Expression under control of the 5' upstream region of the soybean gene was found to be regulated at the level of transcription and followed the correct developmental timing (Jensen et al. 1986). Nodule-specific *trans*-acting factors were shown to interact specifically with defined sequences located within this 5' upstream region (E. Oestergaard Jensen et al., in prep.).

Heat-inducible Genes. By taking 5' upstream sequences from so-called heat shock genes (i.e., genes that are active only after a treatment of diverse organisms—such as plants or insects—at elevated temperatures for about 1 hr), chimeric genes were constructed that are active in transgenic plants after a heat shock treatment but not at normal temperatures (Spena et al. 1985; Spena and Schell 1987).

Targeting Genes for Transport of Foreign Proteins into Chloroplasts

As an alternative to transforming directly foreign genes into a cell compartment, one can exploit a well-known transport mechanism that targets translation products of nuclear genes to the organellar compartments. The natural transport system of the small subunit of rbcS/oxygenase was used for this purpose. During or shortly after translocation, the transit peptide, which facilitates the transport process, is cleaved off from the precursor protein to yield the mature polypeptide. A foreign polypeptide, namely APTII from transposon Tn5, was shown to be transported into chloroplasts of tobacco provided that the transit peptide was fused to the APTII polypeptide (Schreier et al. 1985; Van den Broeck et al. 1985).

It is therefore possible to target foreign proteins for transport into chloroplasts by constructing chimeric genes that will, upon transcription and translation in transgenic plants, produce a fusion protein consisting of a transit peptide sequence at

7

its amino-terminal end fused to the protein targeted to be transported into chloroplasts (Schrier and Schell 1986).

The examples that have been described briefly here clearly indicate that it is possible to use a series of expression vectors to construct chimeric genes that will be expressed in plants at either high or low levels, or induced by environmental factors such as light, temperature, chemicals (e.g., fungal elicitors), or wounding, or expressed only in specific organs such as leaves, seeds, tubers, roots, or flowers. By manipulating proteins to be transported into chloroplasts it might be possible to protect such chloroplasts against the action of herbicides and improve their photosynthetic capacity.

Isolation of Plant Genes by Gene Tagging

Best known in plants through the work of Barbara McClintock (McClintock 1951; Fedoroff 1983), transposable elements, by their insertion, have been cloned and used as probes to isolate genes reversibly mutated (Wienand and Saedler 1987). The time-consuming step in this approach is the genetic analysis of the mutant plants. The molecular isolation of the tagged locus, however, is very straightforward.

This approach was made available to plants for which no transposable elements are known or cloned. When the maize-controlling element *Ac* was tranferred into tobacco by means of a Ti-plasmid vector and shown to excise from its original location in the tDNA and to integrate in the tobacco genome (Baker et al. 1986), by constructing an NPTII gene whose expression is prevented by the insertion of an *Ac* element, a convenient system for the phenotypic assay of *Ac* transposition activity in foreign host plants was developed (Baker et al. 1987).

Agrobacterium-mediated transformation itself, leading to random integration of tDNA segments, is also useful as a gene tag. Some Ti-plasmid vectors have been designed specifically for this purpose (Andre et al. 1986; Koncz et al. 1987b). The potential advantage of tDNA-based tags is that in most transgenic plant cells, the tDNA is inserted at a single locus. The disadvantage, relative to transposable elements, is the lack of reversion of the mutant phenotype, which is the most convenient way to demonstrate that the mutant phenotype is the direct consequence of insertion of the gene tag.

Gene Transfer as an Additional Tool in Plant Breeding

Although transgenic plants actually expressing chimeric genes were first reported in 1983, we are already witnessing the prac-

8

tical use of these methods for agriculturally relevant plant breeding. Not surprisingly, all of these early examples have to do with the transfer and expression of single genes, and several of these are derived from bacterial genes. Probably the most advanced examples involve genes protecting crop plants against nonselective herbicides (Shah et al. 1986; De Block et al. 1987). Other examples are relevant for insect control (Vaeck et al. 1987) or tolerance to viral infections (Powell-Abel et al. 1986). These are but the first examples of major applications, but they demonstrate the validity and the potential of this approach. It might be argued that the host range of *Agrobacterium* is limited and that some of the most important crops, such as cereals, are not amenable to the described gene-transfer techniques. However, in the near future, techniques will be available to introduce genes into most any crop, including the major cereals.

It appears that some of these techniques will be fairly simple and perhaps somewhat mundane when compared to the refined mechanism used by *Agrobacterium* itself. Indeed, direct injection, with a hypodermic needle, of DNA coding for a selectable marker gene (*aptII*) into the tillers of rye just underneath a developing influorescence apparently led to the uptake of the DNA in the genome of developing germ cells. From among 3000 seeds obtained from a few hundred injected plants, 3 independent transgenic plants were obtained that contained and expressed the transferred kanamycin-resistant gene (De la Pena et al. 1987). An even more direct way to introduce genes into cereals is suggested by the observation that mechanically isolated mature wheat embryos derived from dry seeds are able to take up DNA by imbibition of a DNA solution and express a chimeric NPTII gene transiently. These DNA-treated embryos can readily be cultured into full plants (R. Töpfer et al., in prep.). Whether offspring from plants derived from these DNA-treated embryos have inherited integrated copies of the introduced DNA remains to be determined.

REFERENCES
Andre, D., D. Colau, J. Schell, M. Van Montagu, and J.-P. Hernalsteens. 1986. Gene tagging plants by a T-DNA insertion mutagen that generates APH(3′)II-plant gene fusions. *Mol. Gen. Genet.* **204:** 512.
Baker, B., J. Schell, H. Lörz, and N. Fedoroff. 1986. Transposition of the maize controlling element activator in tobacco. *Proc. Natl. Acad. Sci.* **83:** 4844.

Baker, B., G. Coupland, N. Fedoroff, P. Starlinger, and J. Schell. 1987. Phenotypic assay for excision of the maize controlling element *Ac* in tobacco. *EMBO J.* **6:** 1547.

Bevan, M. 1984. Binary *Agrobacterium* vectors for plant transformation. *Nucleic Acids Res.* **12:** 8711.

Bojsen, K., D. Abildsten, E.O. Jensen, K. Paludan, and K.A. Marcker. 1983. The chromosomal arrangement of six soybean leghemoglobin genes. *EMBO J.* **2:** 1165.

Buchanan-Wollaston, V., J.E. Passiatore, and F. Cannon. 1987. The *mob* and *oriT* mobilization functions of a bacterial plasmid promote its transfer to plants. *Nature* **328:** 172.

Coruzzi, G., R. Broglie, C. Edwards, and N.-H. Chua. 1984. Tissue-specific and light-regulated expression of a pea nuclear gene encoding the small subunit of ribulose-1,5-bisphosphate carboxylase. *EMBO J.* **3:** 1671.

De Block, M., J. Botterman, M. Vandewiele, J. Dockx, C. Thoen, V. Gossele, N. Rao Movva, C. Thompson, M. Van Montagu, and J. Leemans. 1987. Engineering herbicide resistance in plants by expression of a detoxifying enzyme. *EMBO J.* **6:** 2513.

De la Pena, A., H. Lörz, and J. Schell. 1987. Transgenic rye plants obtained by DNA injection into young floral tillers. *Nature* **325:** 274.

Eckes, P., S. Rosahl, J. Schell, and L. Willmitzer. 1986. Isolation and characterization of a light-inducible, organ-specific gene from potato and analysis of its expression after tagging and transfer into tobacco and potato shoots. *Mol. Gen. Genet.* **205:** 14.

Everett, R. and N. Willetts. 1980. Characterization of an *in vivo* system for nicking at the origin of conjugational DNA transfer of the sex factor F.J. *Mol. Biol.* **136:** 129.

Fedoroff, N. 1983. Controlling elements in maize. In *Mobile genetic elements* (ed. J. Shapiro), p. 1. Academic Press, New York.

Fraley, R.T., S.G. Rogers, R.B. Horsch, D.A. Eichholtz, J.S. Flick, C.L. Fink, N.L. Hoffmann, and P.R. Sanders. 1985. The SEV system: A new disarmed Ti plasmid vector system for plant transformation. *Bio/Technology* **3:** 629.

Green, T.R. and C.A. Ryan. 1972. Wound-induced proteinase inhibitors in plant leaves: A possible mechanism against insects. *Science* **175:** 776.

Herrera-Estrella, L., G. Van den Broeck, R. Maenhaut, M. Van Montagu, and J. Schell. 1984. Light-inducible and chloroplast-associated expression of a chimaeric gene introduced into *Nicotiana tabacum* using Ti plasmid vector. *Nature* **310:** 115.

Jefferson, R.A., T.A. Kavanagh, and M.W. Bevan. 1987. GUS fusions: β-glucuronidase as a sensitive and versatile gene fusion marker in higher plants. *EMBO J.* **6:** 3901.

Jensen, J.S., K.A. Marcker, L. Otten, and J. Schell. 1986. Nodule-specific expression of a chimaeric soybean leghaemoglobin gene in transgenic *Lotus corniculatus*. *Nature* **321:** 669.

Kaulen, H., J. Schell, and F. Kreuzaler. 1986. Light induced expression of the chimeric chalcone synthase NPTII gene in tobacco cells. *EMBO J.* **5:** 1.

Keil, M., J. Sanchez-Serrano, J. Schell, and L. Willmitzer. 1986. Primary structure of a proteinase inhibitor II gene from potato (*Solanum tuberosum*). *Nucleic Acids Res.* **14**: 5641.

Koncz, C. and J. Schell. 1986. The promoter of T_L-DNA gene 5 controls the tissue specific expression of chimeric genes carried by a novel type of *Agrobacterium* binary vector. *Mol. Gen. Genet.* **204**: 383.

Koncz, C., O. Olsson, W.H.R. Langridge, J. Schell, and A.A. Szalay. 1987a. Expression and functional assembly of bacterial luciferase in plants. *Proc. Natl. Acad. Sci.* **84**: 131.

Koncz, C., N. Martini, Z. Koncz, O. Olsson, A. Radermacher, A. Szalay, and J. Schell. 1987b. Genetic tools for the analysis of gene expression in plants. In *Tailoring genes for crop improvement* (ed. G. Bruening et al.), p. 197. Plenum Publishing, New York.

Lee, J.S., G.G. Brown, and D.P.S. Verma. 1985. Chromosomal arrangement of leghemoglobin genes in soybean. *Nucleic Acids Res.* **11**: 5541.

McClintock, B. 1951. Chromosome organization and genetic expression. *Cold Spring Harbor Symp. Quant. Biol.* **16**: 13.

Morelli, G., F. Nagy, R.T. Fraley, S.G. Rogers, and N.H. Chua. 1985. A short conserved sequence is involved in the light-inducibility of a gene encoding ribulose 1,5-bisphosphate carboxylase small subunit of pea. *Nature* **315**: 200.

Ow, D.W., K.V. Wood, M. DeLuca, J.R. De Wet, D.R. Helinski, and S.H. Howell. 1986. Transient and stable expression of the firefly luciferase gene in plant cells and transgenic plants. *Science* **234**: 856.

Powell-Abel, P., R.S. Nelson, D.E. Barun, N. Hoffmann, S.G. Rogers, R.T. Fraley, and R.N. Beachy. 1986. Delay of disease development in transgenic plants that express the tobacco mosaic virus coat protein gene. *Science* **232**: 738.

Rosahl, S., P. Eckes, J. Schell, and L. Willmitzer. 1986. Organ-specific gene expression in potato: Isolation and characterization of tuber-specific cDNA sequences. *Mol. Gen. Genet.* **202**: 368.

Ryan, C.A. 1977. Proteolytic enzymes and their inhibitors in plants. *Annu. Rev. Plant Physiol.* **24**: 173.

Sanchez-Serrano, J., R. Schmidt, J. Schell, and L. Willmitzer. 1986. Nucleotide sequence of proteinase inhibitor II encoding cDNA of potato (*Solanum tuberosum*) and its mode of expression. *Mol. Gen. Genet.* **203**: 15.

Sanchez-Serrano, J.J., M. Keil, A. O'Connor, J. Schell, and L. Willmitzer. 1987. Wound-induced expression of a potato proteinase inhibitor II gene in transgenic tobacco plants. *EMBO J.* **6**: 303.

Schreier, P.H. and J. Schell. 1986. Use of chimaeric gene harbouring small subunit transit peptide sequences to study transport in chloroplasts. *Philos. Trans. R. Soc. Lond. B* **313**: 429.

Schreier, P.H., E.A. Seftor, J. Schell, and H.J. Bohnert. 1985. The use of nuclear encoded sequences to direct the light-regulated synthesis and transport of a foreign protein into plant chloroplasts. *EMBO J.* **4**: 25.

Shah, D.M., R.B. Horsch, H.J. Klee, G.M. Kishore, J.A. Winter, N.E. Turner, C.M. Hironake, P.R. Sanders, C.S. Gasser, S. Aykent, N.R. Siegel, S.G. Rogers, and R.T. Fraley. 1986. Engineering herbicide tolerance in transgenic plants. *Science* **233:** 478.

Simpson, J., J. Schell, M. Van Montagu, and L. Herrera-Estrella. 1986. The light-inducible and tissue-specific expression of a pea LHCP gene involves an upstream element combining enhancer- and silencer-like properties. *Nature* **323:** 551.

Simpson, J., M.P. Timko, A.R. Cashmore, J. Schell, M. Van Montagu, and L. Herrera-Estrella. 1985. Light-inducible and tissue-specific expression of a chimaeric gene under control of the 5' -flanking sequence of pea chlorophyll a/b-binding protein gene. *EMBO J.* **4:** 2723.

Spena, A. and J. Schell. 1987. The expression of a heat inducible chimeric gene in transgenic tobacco plants. *Mol. Gen. Genet.* **206:** 436.

Spena, A., R. Hain, U. Ziervogel, H. Saedler, and J. Schell. 1985. Construction of a heat-inducible gene for plants. Demonstration of heat-inducible activity of the *Drosophila hsp70* promoter in plants. *EMBO J.* **4:** 2739.

Stachel, S.E., B. Timmermann, and P. Zambryski. 1986. Generation of single-stranded T-DNA molecules during the initial stages of T-DNA transfer from *Agrobacterium tumefaciens* to plant cells. *Nature* **322:** 706.

Stachel, S.E., E. Messens, M. Van Montagu, and P. Zambryski. 1985. Identification of the signal molecules produced by wounded plant cells that activate T-DNA transfer in *Agrobacterium tumefaciens*. *Nature* **318:** 624.

Timko, M.P., A.P. Kausch, C. Castresana, J. Fassler, L. Herrera-Estrella, G. Van den Broeck, M. Van Montagu, J. Schell, and A.R. Cashmore. 1985. Light regulation of plant gene expression by an enhancer-like element. *Nature* **318:** 579.

Tobin, E.M. and J. Silverthorne. 1985. Light regulation of gene expression in higher plants. *Annu. Rev. Plant Physiol.* **36:** 569.

Vaeck, M., H. Höfte, A. Reynaerts, J. Leemans, M. Van Montagu, and M. Zabeau. 1987. Engineering of insect resistant plants using a *B. thuringiensis* gene. *UCLA Symp. Mol. Cell. Biol. New Ser.* **48:** 355.

Van den Broeck, G., M.P. Timko, A.P. Kausch, A.R. Cashmore, M. Van Montagu, and L. Herrera-Estrella. 1985. Targeting of a foreign protein to chloroplasts by fusion to the transit peptide from the small subunit of ribulose 1,5-bisphosphate carboxylase. *Nature* **313:** 358.

Wang, K., L. Herrera-Estrella, M. Van Montagu, and P. Zambryski. 1984. Right 25-bp terminus sequence of the nopaline T-DNA is essential for and determines direction of DNA transfer from *Agrobacterium* to the plant genome. *Cell* **38:** 455.

Wienand, U. and H. Saedler. 1987. Plant transposable elements: Unique structures for gene tagging and gene cloning. In *Plant gene research IV: Plant DNA infectious agents* (ed. T. Hohn and J. Schell), p. 204. Springer-Verlag, West Germany.

Zambryski, P., H. Joos, C. Genetello, J. Leemans, M. Van Montagu, and J. Schell. 1983. Ti plasmid vector for the introduction of DNA into plant cells without alteration of their normal regeneration capacity. *EMBO J.* **2:** 2143.

Strategies for Practical Gene Transfer into Agriculturally Important Crops

R.B. Horsch, J. Fry, M.A.W. Hinchee, H.J. Klee, S.G. Rogers, and R.T. Fraley

Monsanto Company, St. Louis, Missouri 63198

In the past 4 years, two techniques have been developed for transferring isolated genes into plant cells and regenerating transgenic plants from those cells. One method is based on the capacity of plant protoplasts to incorporate and express exogenous DNA when treated with physical or electrical treatments to permeabilize their membranes. The other method is based on the natural gene transfer capacity of *Agrobacterium tumefaciens*, which can transform cells as well as protoplasts.

In theory, the delivery of exogenous DNA to protoplasts is without host limitation, whereas *A. tumefaciens* has been observed to transform only dicotyledonous species and a few monocots in the lily family. In practice to date, a much broader range of transgenic plants has been produced with *A. tumefaciens*-mediated transformation because it can transform regenerable tissues with relative ease, whereas protoplasts of most species are still relatively difficult or impossible to regenerate. Free DNA delivery to regenerable protoplasts may be the eventual key to transformation of important crops such as corn, wheat, or rice, but because of the practical ease of *A. tumefaciens*-mediated transformation, it is likely to remain the method of choice for routine production of transgenic plants for species within its host range. Recently, the possibility of using *A. tumefaciens* for gene transfer to monocot crops has been raised by the finding that maize streak virus (MSV) can be transferred to maize plants by the technique of agroinfection (Grimsley et al. 1987) and the detection of opines in infected maize seedlings (Graves and Goldman 1986).

Agrobacterium

A. tumefaciens causes crown gall disease by transferring a defined segment of DNA (T-DNA) from its tumor-inducing (Ti)

plasmid into the nuclear genome of cells in an infected wound on many dicotyledonous plants (for recent review, see Nester et al. 1984). The movement of the T-DNA is mediated by genes in another region of the Ti plasmid. These virulence genes (Klee et al. 1983) are not themselves transferred with the T-DNA but act in *trans* to cause the transfer (de Framond et al. 1983; Hoekema et al. 1983). The T-DNA is defined by a 25-base sequence, the border sequence, which is present as a direct repeat outside the ends of the T-DNA (Barker et al. 1983). Recent evidence suggests that the border sequence is the site of specific nicking of the DNA by one of the virulence gene products (Stachel et al. 1986). It has been reported that a bacterial origin of transfer can substitute for the border sequence when compatible mobilization functions are also present (Buchanan-Wollaston et al. 1987). None of the genes or DNA sequences within the T-DNA are required for the transfer process (Garfinkel et al. 1981).

These properties of the *Agrobacterium* DNA transfer system are invaluable for developing a powerful vector system for plant transformation. It is possible to remove all of the original T-DNA that was responsible for the disease and replace it with any DNA, as long as the border sequence is maintained (Zambryski et al. 1983). The DNA is inherently stable once in the plant genome because neither border nor the virulence genes are transferred. Finally, because the borders define a discrete T-DNA segment, the frequency of cotransfer of the entire segment is very high. This means that your favorite genes are usually transferred along with the selectable marker used to identify the transformed cells or plants.

To harness this mechanism, shuttle vectors have been designed that can replicate in *Escherichia coli*, where recombinant manipulations are easily handled, and then be transferred into *A. tumefaciens* in preparation for transfer into plants. There are two basic modes of maintenance of the shuttle vectors in *Agrobacterium*: either by integration into the Ti plasmid by recombination at a region of DNA homology (Comai et al. 1983; Fraley et al. 1983; Zambryski et al. 1983) or by autonomous replication in *trans* to the Ti plasmid (An et al. 1984; Bevan 1984; Klee et al. 1985). The former type of vector is referred to as a *cis* or integrating vector, whereas the latter is called a *trans* or binary vector. In most cases, they accomplish the same goals of shuttling genes from *E. coli* to *A. tumefaciens* in a T-DNA package that can then be transferred to plants. The most important feature of a vector is the selectable marker for recognition of transformed plant cells.

Selectable Markers

Because only a small proportion of cells are transformed by *A. tumefaciens*, it is important to have a selectable marker to permit growth of the transformed cells and suppress growth of wild-type cells. The first marker to be used was the neomycin phosphotransferase gene from *E. coli*. This gene has been used successfully in many systems, including mammalian cells, fungi, and *Dictyostelium*. In solancious plants such as petunia and tobacco, it provides an excellent, unambiguous selectable marker. The features of a good selectable marker are (1) high-level resistance of the transformed cells to concentrations of the drug that completely inhibit wild-type growth, and (2) efficient selectability of rare transformants from a large excess of inhibited wild-type cells that surround them. Kanamycin-inhibited petunia cells do not appear to interfere with the growth of resistant cells in any way and may actually facilitate their growth by acting as a nurse tissue. Other selectable markers include genes conferring resistance to methotrexate (Eichholtz et al. 1987) or hygromycin (Lloyd et al. 1986). A number of herbicide resistance genes have been developed recently that also can be used as selectable markers.

Leaf Disk Transformation

The simple and powerful interface between *A. tumefaciens* and plant cells is illustrated by the leaf disk transformation system (Horsch et al. 1985), where gene transfer, selection, and regeneration are coupled together in an efficient process. Any responsive explant can be used instead of leaf disks. Although the technique is most easily practiced with tobacco, it has been applied to a number of other species (Table 1).

Position effects, that is, effects of the surrounding DNA or chromatin structure, result in differences in expression of the T-DNA genes in different transformants. The extreme of this is complete loss of expression during differentiation of the plantlet. This occurred in about one quarter to one third of the shoots that grew initially in the presence of 300 μg/ml kanamycin. One possible reason for failure to select against these escapes is that the kanamycin is not a good herbicide, and shoots can continue growth in its presence once they are large enough. It is usually necessary to screen several indepen-

Table 1 Transgenic Plants Produced with *A. tumefaciens*-mediated Transformation

Species	Reference
Nicotiana plumbaginifolia	Horsch et al. (1984)
Petunia	Horsch et al. (1985)
Tobacco	DeBlock et al. (1984)
Tomato	McCormick et al. (1986)
Potato	Shahin and Simpson (1986)
Lettuce	Michelmore et al. (1987)
Poplar	Fillatti et al. (1987)
Arabidopsis thaliana	Lloyd et al. (1986)
Medicago varia	Deak et al. (1986)
Flax	Basiran et al. (1987)
Brassica napus	Fry et al. (1987)
Sunflower	Everett et al. (1987)
Cotton	Umbeck et al. (1987)

dent transgenic plants to identify the best expression of your favorite gene, which sometimes but not always is correlated with the expression of the selectable marker.

Inheritance

Progeny usually inherit the T-DNA according to Mendelian rules for dominant genes. In cases where there is only one T-DNA, selfed progeny show a 3:1 ratio for nopaline or kanamycin resistance, whereas backcrossed progeny show a 1:1 ratio. This is also true for multiple T-DNAs that are present in a tandem array where they are all genetically linked. In a few cases, there are multiple T-DNAs, some of which are unlinked. In these cases, selfed ratios are usually 15:1 (two unlinked loci) or higher (three or more unlinked loci). In nearly all cases, the selected and unselected markers on a single T-DNA are coinherited.

The T-DNA thus becomes a permanent, stable part of the genome of transgenic plants and behaves just as the other endogenous genes (Wallroth et al. 1986). The availability of plants with T-DNA inserts mapped in chromosomal locations brings a valuable new tool to plant genetics. These transformants have a marker that is scored easily; it can be used to map new mutants and a selectable chromosome tag that might facilitate breeding or selection of interesting genes nearby.

Host Range of *Agrobacterium*

A. tumefaciens has been shown to transform a wide range of dicotyledonous species and a few monocots in the lily family

(De Cleene and De Lay 1976). Two lines of evidence have been published that are suggestive of a compatibility between *A. tumefaciens* and corn. In the study by Grimsley et al. (1987), *A. tumefaciens* was used to introduce MSV into corn plants by a technique called agroinfection. This demonstrated a virulence gene- and border-gene-dependent transfer of MSV DNA from the T-DNA of *A. tumefaciens* into corn plants, resulting in a systemic infection. It should thus be a very sensitive assay of gene transfer because a single event could produce the systemic infection. It does not prove integration of DNA into the corn genome or address practical issues related to germ-line access by cells that may be transformed.

The second line of evidence was published by Graves and Goldman (1986), where they detected nopaline or octopine in tissues of maize seedlings after infection with nopaline or octopine strains of *A. tumefaciens*. These studies are suggestive but not conclusive because of the undependable nature of opine production or opine-like substances in tissues of various plant species, including tissues known not to be transformed (Christou et al. 1986).

Thus, it remains unclear whether *A. tumefaciens* is capable of stable gene transfer to crops such as corn. Further analysis and better assay methods should provide a definite answer within the next year. It still remains to be seen whether *A. tumefaciens* can be engineered to transform species such as corn by modification of attachment functions, induction, or alterations to the virulence genes, or other modifications of the bacterium or coculture conditions.

REFERENCES

An, G., B. Watson, S. Stachel, M. Gordon, and E. Nester. 1984. New cloning vehicles for transformation of higher plants. *EMBO J.* **4:** 277.

Barker, R., K. Idler, D. Thompson, and J. Kemp. 1983. Nucleotide sequence of the T-DNA region from the *Agrobacterium tumefaciens* octopine Ti plasmid pTi15955. *Plant Mol. Biol.* **2:** 335.

Basiran, N., P. Armitage, R.J. Scott, and J. Draper. 1987. Genetic transformation of flax (*Linum usitataissimum*) by *Agrobacterium tumefaciens*: Regeneration of transformed shoots via a callus phase. *Plant Cell Rep.* **6:** 396.

Bevan, M. 1984. *Agrobacterium* vectors for plant transformation. *Nucleic Acids Res.* **12:** 8711.

Buchanan-Wollaston, V., J.E. Passiatore, and F. Cannon. 1987. The mob and oriT mobilization functions of a bacterial plasmid promote its transfer to plants. *Nature* **328:** 172.

Christou, P., S.G. Platt, and M.C. Ackerman. 1986. Opine synthesis in wild-type plant tissue. *Plant Physiol.* **82:** 218.

Comai, I., C. Schilling-Cordaro, A. Mergia, and C. Houck. 1983. A new technique for genetic engineering of *Agrobacterium* Ti plasmid. *Plasmid* **10:** 21.

Deak, M., G.B. Kiss, C. Koncz, and D. Dudits. 1986. Transformation of *Medicago* by *Agrobacterium* mediated gene transfer. *Plant Cell Rep.* **5:** 97.

DeBlock, M., L. Herrera-Estrella, M. Van Montagu, J. Schell, and P. Zambryski. 1984. Expression of foreign genes in regenerated plants and their progeny. *EMBO J.* **3:** 1681.

De Cleene, M. and J. De Lay. 1976. The host range of crown gall. *Bot. Rev.* **42:** 389.

deFrammond, A., K. Barton, and M.D. Chilton. 1983. Mini-Ti: A new vector strategy for plant genetic engineering. *Bio/Technology* **1:** 262.

Eichholtz, D.A., S.G. Rogers, R.B. Horsch, H.J. Klee, M. Hayford, N.L. Hoffman, S.B. Braford, C. Fink, J. Flick, K.M. O'Connell, and R.T. Fraley. 1987. Expression of mouse dihydrofolate reductase gene confers methotrexate resistance in transgenic petunia plants. *Somatic Cell Mol. Genet.* **13:** 67.

Everett, N.P., K.E.P. Robinson, and D. Mascarenhas. 1987. Genetic engineering of sunflower (*Helianthus annuus L.*) Bio/technology (in press).

Fillatti, J.J., J. Sellmer, B. McCown, B. Haissig, and L. Comai. 1987. *Agrobacterium* mediated transformation and regeneration of poplar. *Mol. Gen. Genet.* **206:** 192.

Fraley, R.T., S.G. Rogers, R.B. Horsch, P.R. Sanders, J.S. Flick, S.P. Adams, M.L. Bittner, L.A. Brand, C.L. Fink, J.S. Fry, G.R. Galluppi, S.B. Goldberg, N.L. Hoffmann, and S.C. Woo. 1983. Expression of bacterial genes in plant cells. *Proc. Natl. Acad. Sci.* **80:** 4803.

Fry, J., A. Barnason, and R.B. Horsch. 1987. Transformation of *Brassica napus* with *Agrobacterium tumefaciens* based vectors. *Plant Cell Rep.* **6:** 321.

Garfinkel, D., R. Simpson, L. Ream, F. White, M. Gordon, and E. Nester. 1981. Genetic analysis of crown gall: Fine structure map of the T-DNA by site-directed mutagenesis. *Cell* **27:** 143.

Graves, A.C.F. and S.L. Goldman. 1986. The transformation of Zea mays seedlings with *Agrobacterium tumefaciens:* Detection of T-DNA specific enzymes activities. *Plant Mol. Biol.* **7:** 43.

Grimsley, N., T. Hohn, J.W. Davies, and B. Hohn. 1987. *Agrobacterium*-mediated delivery of infectious maize streak virus into maize plants. *Nature* **325:** 177.

Hoekema, A., P. Hirsch, P. Hooykaas, and R. Schilperoort. 1983. A binary plant vector strategy based on separation of vir- and T-region of the *Agrobacterium tumefaciens* Ti-plasmid. *Nature* **303:** 179.

Horsch, R.B., R.T. Fraley, S.G. Rogers, P.R. Sanders, A. Lloyd, and N. Hoffmann. 1984. Inheritance of functional foreign genes in plants. *Science* **223:** 496.

Horsch, R.B., J. Fry, N.L. Hoffmann, M. Wallroth, D. Eichholtz, S.G.

Rogers, and R.T. Fraley. 1985. A simple and general method for tranferring genes into plants. *Science* **227**: 1229.

Klee, H.J., M.F. Yanofsky, and E.W. Nester. 1985. Vectors for transformation of higher plants. *Bio/Technology* **3**: 637.

Klee, H., F. White, V. Iyer, M. Gordon, and E. Nester. 1983. Mutational analysis of the virulence region of an *Agrobacterium tumefaciens* Ti plasmid. *J. Bacteriol.* **153**: 878.

Lloyd, A.M., A.R. Barnason, S.G. Rogers, M.C. Byrne, R.T. Fraley, and R.B. Horsch. 1986. Transformation of *Arabidopsis thaliana* with *Agrobacterium tumefaciens* using a gene conferring hygromycin resistance. *Science* **234**: 464.

McCormick, S., J. Niedermeyer, J. Fry, A. Barnason, R. Horsch, and R. Fraley. 1986. Leaf disc transformation of cultivated tomato (*L. esculentum*) using *Agrobacterium tumefaciens*. *Plant Cell Rep.* **5**: 81.

Michelmore, R.W., E. Marsh, S. Seely, and B. Landry. 1987. Transformation of lettuce (*Lactuca sativa*) mediated by *Agrobacterium tumefaciens*. *Plant Cell Rep.* (in press).

Nester, E., M. Gordone, R. Amasino, and M. Yanofsky. 1984. Crown gall: A molecular and physiological analysis. *Annu. Rev. Plant. Physiol.* **35**: 387.

Shahin, E. and R. Simpson. 1986. Gene transfer system for potato. *Hortic. Sci.* **21**: 1199.

Stachel, S.E., B. Timmerman, and P. Zambryski. 1986. Generation of single-stranded T-DNA molecules during the initial stages of T-DNA transfer from *Agrobacterium tumefaciens* to plant cells. *Natutre* **322**: 796.

Umbeck, R., G. Johnson, K. Barton, and W. Swain. 1987. Genetically transformed cotton (Gossypium hirsutum L.) plants. *Bio/Technology* **5**: 263.

Wallroth, M., A.G.M. Gerats, S.G. Rogers, R.T. Fraley, and R.B. Horsch. 1986. Chromosomal localization of foreign genes in Petunia hybrida. *Mol. Gen. Genet.* **202**: 6.

Zambryski, P., H. Joos, C. Genetello, J. Leemans, M. Van Montagu, and J. Schell. 1983. Ti plasmid vector for the introduction of DNA into plants cells without alteration of their normal regeneration capacity. *EMBO J.* **2**: 2143.

Maize Transformation via Microprojectile Bombardment

A. Weissinger, D. Tomes, S. Maddock, M. Fromm, and J. Sanford

Pioneer Hi-Bred International, Inc.
Johnston, Iowa 50131

An efficient technology for the genetic transformation of maize is required both to facilitate genetic studies and to allow the introduction of agriculturally useful genes. Plant transformation has become routine for some species (Fraley et al. 1986) but remains an elusive goal for most monocotyledonous species. Significant progress has been made in this area with techniques such as electroporation (Fromm et al. 1985) and calcium phosphate coprecipitation (Lorz et al. 1985). It is now a relatively ordinary procedure to achieve "transient" expression in protoplasts from cultured maize cells, although little success has been achieved in attempts to advance the technology to intact cells. Several laboratories have also been able to recover stably transformed callus from electroporated protoplasts (Fromm et al. 1986) and, in one instance (C. Rhodes, pers. comm.), plants have been regenerated. Protoplast manipulations, especially regeneration from protoplasts, remain unreliable and difficult.

Most alternative technologies for maize transformation suffer similar limitations. DNA delivery via microinjection of maize cells has been accomplished successfully (Crossway et al. 1986; A. Crossway, pers. comm.). The technique is very time consuming and highly technical, however, so that the number of potentially transformed cells that can be produced is relatively small. This constraint probably limits microinjection to single-cell systems in which the probability of regeneration is very high.

Transformations of maize by *Agrobacterium* species would be extremely useful. Host specificity of the bacterium, however, has been a major impediment to successful application of the technique to most monocots (Fraley et al. 1986). Some progress has been made in achieving *Agrobacterium* infection in maize seedlings, suggesting that *Agrobacterium*-mediated transformation may eventually be applicable to maize transformation (S. Goldman, pers. comm.).

Because of the limitations inherent in other technologies, we became interested in microprojectile bombardment for delivery of transforming DNAs into intact, potentially totipotent maize cells. In this procedure, developed by J.C. Sanford and coworkers (Klein et al. 1987), microscopic (~1-µm) tungsten particles (microprojectiles), associated with plasmid DNA, are accelerated to approximately 400 meters per second in a "particle gun" apparatus. These very dense particles thus acquire sufficient kinetic energy to penetrate intact cell walls and membranes.

A chimeric chloramphenicol acetyl transferase (CAT) gene construction was successfully delivered into epidermis cells of *Allium cepa* using this technique. Expression of the introduced gene could be detected, demonstrating that the DNA delivered in this fashion was available for subsequent transcription. It also showed that treated cells could tolerate the trauma of bombardment.

Microprojectile Bombardment of Maize
Suspension Cultures

Our first step in the adaptation of microprojectile bombardment to maize was the treatment of suspension culture cells derived from maize cultivar Black Mexican Sweet (BMS) (generously prorvided by V. Walbot). For complete details, see Klein et al. (1988). These smaller, spheroidal cells, often in small clusters, were a very difficult target compared with the larger, planar *Allium* cells for which the procedure was originally perfected.

To maximize the number of cells exposed to bombardment, clusters were separated by passage through a 710-µm mesh sieve prior to treatment. Masses of these cells (100 mg) were bombarded with 1.2-µm microprojectiles coated with plasmid DNA, as described previously (Klein et al. 1987). Single-bombardment treatments delivered about 350 ng of transforming DNA in each bombardment. Vectors used contained a CAT gene construction with the cauliflower mosaic virus 35S promoter (CaMV 35S) and nopaline synthase 3' region (NOS 3') (pCaMVCN), or a similar plasmid (pCaMVI$_1$CN) in which a segment of the maize Adh1 intron 1, inserted between promoter and structural gene sequences, functioned as an enhancer of gene expression (these constructions will be described in detail in J. Callis et al., in prep.).

Cells bombarded with pCaMVCN did not express detectable levels of CAT, 96 hours following bombardment. However, those cells treated with the enhanced pCaMVI₁CN expressed levels of CAT activity comparable to that produced in similar masses of protoplasts transformed with this vector. CAT levels as high as 57 units per gram of soluble protein were observed in replicated experiments. Similar experiments were attempted in the embryogenic suspension cultures 3-86-17 and 13-217 (for details of the preparation of these cultures, see Klein et al. 1988). These cultures, unlike the older BMS suspensions, retain the ability to regenerate whole plants. Such embryogenic cells are an even more formidable subject for microprojectile bombardment, however, because of their very small size and the growth of cells in large aggregates in culture. These bombardments resulted in CAT expression at levels of approximately 3 units per gram of soluble protein, substantially below levels observed in BMS tissue treated under identical conditions.

Several parameters of the bombardment process were examined to determine which affected transformation. These included osmotic adjustment, which might reduce cell disruption during bombardment; protection of cells from desiccation with a covering of oil during bombardment; variation in microprojectile diameter to enhance transformation of smaller cells; and increased DNA load on microprojectiles. All proved ineffective, although results from particle diameter experiments and DNA loading experiments were equivocal, requiring further study. Increasing the number of bombardments on a single tissue mass from one to three bombardments proved especially useful, increasing expression level fourfold. This is interesting and somewhat unexpected, because it indicates that treated cells can tolerate repeated bombardment. This offers the possibility of greatly enhanced transformation through heavier bombardment, which was originally expected to be lethal to the treated cells.

We were also able to demonstrate that high levels of expression are not achieved until about 72 hours following bombardment. This is an important finding because it may define proper timing of selection. It is also useful for transient gene expression studies.

Advancement toward Stable Transformation

Results described above were obtained from suspension culture cells harvested for CAT assay from 24 to 96 hours following bombardment. Several experiments were subsequently conducted in which the chimeric CAT plasmid pCaMVI$_1$CN was combined in equal quantities with the vector pCaMVI$_1$HygN, which carries a chimeric hygromycin phosphatase (HPT) gene associated with the CaMV 35S promoter, Adh1 intron 1 enhancer sequence, and NOS 3' regions. Embryogenic (3-86-17 and 3-217) suspension cultures bombarded with this mixture were found to produce levels of CAT enzyme activity 12 days after plating on selective levels of hygromycin, which were equivalent to levels observed at 72 hours. Although these cultures have not yet yielded proven stable transformants, these data do suggest that bombarded cells can survive and express alien genes for protracted periods. The data also suggest that cotransformation via this technique may be a useful strategy for transformation employing nonselectable agronomic genes.

Progress toward recovery of maize plants transformed by microprojectile bombardment continues. Introduction of a chimeric β-glucuronidase (GUS) gene construction, followed by histochemical staining (Jefferson et al. 1986), has allowed the study and improvement of bombardment parameters by providing direct evidence of the physical effects of each factor tested. Suspension culture conditions are under study to optimize timing of bombardment with respect to cell cycle. Cotransformation using both GUS and neomycin phosphotransferase (kanamycin resistance) constructions appears to be effective. Bombardment of newly initiated callus tissue and other target tissues is now being tested and shows considerable promise, providing for high probabilities of plant regeneration not commonly obtainable in other types of cultures.

DISCUSSION

Microprojectile bombardment has been applied successfully to both nonregenerable and embryogenic suspension cultures of maize. Subsequent studies have revealed several parameters that affect transformation efficiency, and the technology is now being extended to other tissue sources, such as embryogenic callus. As it is now engendered, microprojectile bombardment is a rapid and efficient technique that offers a useful alternative to electroporation for transient gene expression studies in maize.   Recovery of transformed maize plants produced by means of this unusual technology has become a real possibility.

REFERENCES

Crossway, A., J.V. Oakes, J.M. Irvine, B. Ward, V. Knauf, and C.K. Shewmaker. 1986. Integration of foreign DNA following microinjection of tobacco mesophyll protoplasts. *Mol. Gen. Genet.* **202:** 79.

Fraley, R.T., R.B. Rogers, and R.B. Horsch. 1986. Genetic transformation in higher plants. *Crit. Rev. Plant Sci.* **4:** 1.

Fromm, M., L.P. Taylor, and V. Walbot. 1985. Expression of genes transferred into monocot and dicot plant cells by electroporation. *Proc. Natl. Acad. Sci.* **82:** 5824.

————. 1986. Stable transformation of maize after gene expression by electroporation. *Nature* **319:** 791.

Jefferson, R.A., S.M. Burgess, and D. Hirsh. 1986. β-Glucuronidase from *Escherichia coli* as a gene-fusion marker. *Proc. Natl. Acad. Sci.* **83:** 447.

Klein, T.M., E.D. Wolf, R. Wu, and J.C. Stanford. 1987. High velocity microprojectiles for delivering nucleic acids into living cells. *Nature* **327:** 70.

Klein, T.M., M. Fromm, A. Weissinger, D. Tomes, S. Schaaf, M. Sletten, and J.C. Sanford. 1988. Transfer of foreign genes into intact maize cells using high velocity microprojectiles. *Proc. Natl. Acad. Sci.* (in press).

Lorz, H., B. Baker, and J. Schell. 1985. Gene transfer to cereal cells mediated by protoplast transformation. *Mol. Gen. Genet.* **199:** 178.

Use of RFLP Analysis to Identify Genes Involved in Complex Traits of Agronomic Importance

T. Helentjaris

Molecular Biology Group, Native Plants, Inc., Salt Lake City
Utah 84108

Although our progress in the technology involved in the actual transfer of DNA into plants has improved significantly over the last few years, our current list of genes to eventually transfer is still limited. Genes for herbicide tolerance, resistance to insect feeding, and viral disease were all originally targeted, as it was known that introduction of a novel, single gene, not found in the target species, could accomplish the desired effect. Although these traits are certainly useful commerically, they would not top the list cited by plant breeders as their primary goals. Yield, maturity, standability, and stress tolerances are invariably some of the most important considerations in the improvement of any cultivar, but these have been essentially disregarded by most researchers as impractical targets for genetic engineering due to their complex inheritance, implying the involvement of many genes.

It is a frequent assumption in quantitative genetics for theoretical considerations that a quantitative trait is the result of cumulative actions of large numbers of genes, each individual gene itself contributing an insignificant effect. If this were strictly true, genetic engineering of one or a few genes to improve such a trait would be necessarily doomed to failure. For the last several years at Native Plants, Inc. (NPI), we have been exploring the application of restriction fragment length polymorphism (RFLP) analysis to problems in plant genetics and breeding, with particular attention to dissection of quantitative traits (see Nienhuis et al. 1987). Our studies with a number of traits, such as soluble solids in tomato and plant height and grain yield in corn, indicate that in each case, relatively few loci can be identified that individually have major effects upon these complex traits. Our results would suggest that although a large number of genes can have an important effect upon complex traits if their function is significantly disturbed, most of these genes probably have little effect upon the total variance for that trait when selected germ plasm is considered. In this latter case, a comparatively small number of genes can often account for a relatively large amount of the total variance. Because variation in gene expression of only a smaller number of genes can impact these traits significantly, it would suggest that engineering their expression could prove sufficient to effect improvement of these "quantitative" traits.

If one is to improve a commercially important but complex trait through genetic engineering of one or a few genes, the most productive approach would be to utilize genes already involved in this process but to alter their levels of expression or function in a direction shown to be beneficial. Ideally, this alteration might produce variation that is beyond what is naturally available. To be a viable candidate for such an approach, several criteria need to be met. First, the gene should exhibit a major impact upon the desired trait. Second, the gene should be dominant, or at least additive in its gene action, so that when introduced into a "normal" background, its effect will be realized. Finally, the gene should be simple in its function and not be dependent upon the addition of other genes to the target background.

RFLP analysis of complex traits can supply us with these types of information and, hence, may furnish a means of identifying those endogenous genes that would impact complex traits most significantly. Major quantitative trait loci (QTL) can be localized along the chromosome through correlation of the genotypes of multiple, mapped RFLP loci with portions of the phenotypic variance. The impact of an individual locus on the total plant phenotype can also be ascertained through determining the amount of variance accounted for by it. Those that can account for the greatest amount of variance would, by definition, cause the greatest impact on whole plant phenotype and, hence, be the most obvious candidates for engineering. Gene action can also be determined as being of a recessive, additive, or dominant nature; only those exhibiting an additive or dominant action would be considered for further study. Finally, through multivariate analysis, it can be determined whether the variance accounted for by the QTL is independent of other loci for its effect or whether other loci would be required to obtain the desired effect.

Currently, genes are identified as candidates likely to affect multigenic traits by either physiological or biochemical analyses of pathways that would logically seem to be involved in the trait of interest. We see the RFLP strategy as an alternative approach on the basis of genetic analysis and dissection of the whole plant phenotype. It must be remembered, however, that rather than pinpointing identified genes, we are simply recognizing areas of the genome that account for some measurable amount of the total variance, sometimes on the order of only a few percent. To clone the responsible gene residing within this area is not trivial. One scenario we envision is to correlate our QTL with a known extreme phenotype mutant that could be cloned by conventional methods, such as transposable element insertion mutagenesis or differential cDNA cloning. If the position of the RFLP markers is closely correlated with the conventional linkage map for that species, one could compare the locations of the QTL with mutants with similar phenotypes. Efforts could then be directed toward confirming that both phenotypes represented the results of different expressions of the same gene.

This points out some of the limitations of this strategy. Some species may have a poorly developed linkage map; hence, one may not be able to correlate the QTL with any clonable locus. Alternatively, even in a species with a well-developed map, no known mutant may yet be mapped near the location of the QTL. Finally, this approach is very amenable to the use of transposons to clone the extreme phenotype allele; other strategies may not prove as workable. Species without a practical transposon system may have to be reconsidered.

Obviously, some species and traits may prove to be better targets than others for this approach; in many respects, corn would be an ideal example containing an excellent conventional and RFLP map and several functional transposable element systems. In one actual example of this approach in progress, it was determined, in collaborative studies between C. Stuber and M. Edwards of North Carolina State University and ourselves (unpubl.) that several QTL could be detected with marker loci in maize that had a significant impact on plant height. One locus was found near the centromere of chromosome 9, which could account individually for at least 27% of the variance for this trait (Helentjaris and Shattuck-Eidens 1987). Comparison of this location of the QTL with that of more extreme phenotype mutants on the conventional genetic linkage map showed that it was extremely close to a known GA-biosynthetic dwarf mutant, *d3*. This QTL was shown to be recessive in gene action for shortened stature, and by measuring both internode distance and number of nodes in a segregating population, it was also determined that its effect was exerted primarily by the shortening of the internodal distance. Both of these facts are also true of *d3*, and it is tantalizing to think that both may represent the results of differential gene expression at the same locus. Further efforts are now in progress to confirm the correlation of this QTL with a GA-biosynthetic defect and to clone the *d3* locus through transposable element insertion mutagenesis.

Obtainment of this clone would allow us to confirm that differential gene expression at a single locus could result in an extreme phenotype mutant, as well as function as a major QTL in a quantitative trait. It would verify the strategy of cloning QTL of commercially important traits by relating them to extreme phenotypic loci. With clones for such loci, we believe it will then be possible to impact complex traits significantly through genetic engineering of one or only a few loci and obtain improvements beyond that available through conventional plant breeding.

REFERENCES

Helentjaris, T. and D. Shattuck-Eidens. 1987. A strategy for pinpointing and cloning major genes involved in quantitative traits. *Maize Genet. Coop. News Lett.* **61**: 88.

Nienhuis, J., T. Helentjaris, M. Slocum, B. Ruggero, and A. Schaefer. 1987. Restriction fragment length polymorphism analysis of loci associated with insect resistance in tomato. *Crop Sci.* **27**: 797.

Plant Defense Gene Regulation

C.J. Lamb, M. Dron, S.D. Clouse, R.A. Dixon, and M.A. Lawton

Plant Biology Laboratory, Salk Institute for Biological Studies
San Diego, California 92138

Plants respond to microbial attack or mechanical damage by elaboration of a number of inducible defense responses, including synthesis of phytoalexins, deposition of lignin, accumulation of cell-wall hydroxyproline-rich glycoproteins, and increases in the activity of hydrolytic enzymes. Such responses can also be induced by glycan and glycoprotein elicitors obtained from fungal cell walls and culture fluids. Disease resistance is an active process, dependent on host RNA and protein synthesis. Recent studies have shown that fungal elicitor or pathogen attack causes massive changes in the pattern of host RNA synthesis, including transcriptional activation of defense genes encoding the lytic enzymes chitinase and glucanase, cell-wall hydroxyproline-rich glycoproteins, and enzymes involved in the synthesis of lignin and phytoalexins (Cramer et al. 1985; Lamb et al. 1987; Lawton and Lamb 1987). Accumulation of defense gene transcripts leads to marked stimulation of the synthesis of the encoded proteins and expression of the corresponding defense responses.

These observations focus attention on the molecular mechanisms regulating transcription of defense genes as an early component in the sequence of events between microbial recognition and erection of plant defenses. Genes that regulate activiation of plant defenses represent key targets for manipulation by gene transfer to enhance the natural resistance of crops to disease. We describe here some recent studies on the molecular mechanisms that regulate bean (*Phaseolus vulgaris*) defense genes encoding chalcone synthase (CHS), which catalyzes the stepwise condensation of 4-coumaroyl-CoA with three acetate units from malonyl-CoA to give naringenin chalcone. This is the first and key regulatory reaction of a branch of phenylpropanoid metabolism specific for the synthesis of isoflavonoid phytoalexins in legumes, as well as flavonoid pigments and UV protectants, which are ubiquitous in higher plants. Elicitor stimulates *chs* transcription in bean cells within 5 minutes, leading to a rapid, marked, but transient, accumulation of CHS mRNA with maximum levels after 3–4 hours correlated with the onset of phytoalexin synthesis (Lawton and Lamb 1987).

Transient Assay of *chs* Promoter

To analyze *chs* promoter function, the expression of a chimeric gene comprising the 5′-flanking region of *chs*-λ15 fused with the coding sequences of chloramphenicol acetyltransferase (*cat*) and the 3′-flanking sequences of the nopaline synthase gene (*nos*) was examined following electroporation into protoplasts derived from suspension-cultured soybean (*Glycine max*) cells. *chs*-λ15 is one of six *chs* genes in the bean genome and encodes a major elicitor-induced *chs* transcript (Ryder et al. 1987). As reported recently for parsley protoplasts (Dangl et al. 1987), in our hands soybean protoplasts respond to elicitor in a manner that closely resembles the response of the suspension-cultured cells from which the protoplasts were derived with respect to (1) the kinetics for accumulation of transcripts encoded by endogenous defense genes and (2) appearance of phenylpropanoid products.

Elicitor treatment of electroporated protoplasts caused a marked increase in expression of the chimeric gene within 3 hours, whereas in untreated controls there was no significant change in CAT activity in this period (Fig. 1). In contrast, elicitor did not modulate CAT activity in protoplasts electroporated with a chimeric gene comprising the promoter of the murine histone H_4 gene fused with the *cat-nos* reporter cassette. The chimeric *chs-cat-nos* gene was expressed transiently with maximum levels 3 hours after addition of elicitor, followed by a decay to relatively low levels at 6 and 24 hours after elicitation.

These data indicate that sequences to −326 of the *chs*-λ15 gene are sufficient to confer elicitor regulation in soybean protoplasts. To delineate further the sequences involved in elicitor regulation, the effects of a series of 5′ deletions on expression of the chimeric gene were examined. Deletion to −173 markedly increased the basal level of CAT activity in soybean protoplasts, and moreover, caused a striking increase in the response to elicitor. In contrast, further deletion to −130 reduced both basal and induced expression back to about the

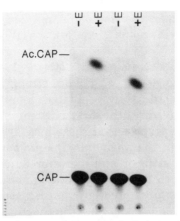

Figure 1 Elicitor induction of the expression of a chimeric *chs-cat-nos* gene in electroporated protoplasts. (−E) Untreated control; (+E) 3 hr after elicitor treatment. Data from two independently electroporated and induced replicates are presented. (CAP) Chloramphenicol (CAT substrate); (Ac.CAP) acetyl-chloramphenicol (CAT product).

same respective levels observed with the entire promoter. Deletion to −72 reduced expression in both elicitor-treated and control protoplasts to the same basal level observed with a construct in which the TATA box (−29 to −21) was deleted (−19).

DISCUSSION

We conclude that there are at least two elements in the 5′-flanking region of *chs*-λ15 that affect the level of expression in protoplasts: a silencer upstream of −173 and an elicitor-regulated activator between −173 and the TATA box. Because deletions beyond −130 in the 3′ direction disrupted elicitor regulation by inhibition of induction rather than by elevation of basal expression, we propose that the activator functions as a positive *cis*-acting element. This functional analysis is consistent with the pattern of sites hypersensitive to DNase-I digestion in *chs* genes. Three such sites, which denote local opening of chromatin structure associated with binding of regulatory proteins, are found in the proximal region of the promoter in nuclei from elicitor-treated but not control cells. In contrast, the upstream silencer region contains sites that show pronounced DNase-I hypersensitivity in nuclei from uninduced as well as elicited cells. Functional analysis of the nested 5′ deletions does not indicate whether the silencer is elicitor regulated, although synergistic interaction between positive and negative elicitor-regulated elements would provide a plausible "gain" mechanism for the very rapid, marked, but transient, activation of defense genes from low basal levels in elicitor-treated cells.

Only two sequence elements, −243 to −194 and −74 to −52, in the 5'-flanking region of CHS are strongly conserved in the promoter of a coordinately regulated gene encoding phenylalanine ammonia–lyase, the first enzyme of phenylpropanoid biosynthesis. We propose that these motifs, which are similarly arranged within the phenylalanine ammonia–lyase promoter, have roles in silencer and activator function, respectively. Construction of point mutations and chimeric promoters is in progress to define more precisely the silencer and activator sequence elements and to examine the function of the silencer in elicitor regulation.

Although transient expression of genes introduced into protoplasts has been demonstrated in several cases, the only previous report of appropriate regulation in response to an external cue is the stimulation of expression of a chimeric *adh-cat-nos* gene in electroporated maize protoplasts induced by oxygen depletion (Walker et al. 1987). It appears that the signal transduction mechanisms for activation of stress-induced genes such as *adh* (alcohol dehydrogenase) and *chs* remain functional during protoplast isolation and culture. The transient assays for defense gene activation in electroporated protoplasts described here now allows precise identification of the *cis*-acting elements for elicitor regulation which will, in turn, facilitate the isolation of the corresponding *trans*-acting regulatory proteins and molecular cloning of the regulatory genes. This approach should open up novel strategies for engineering-enhanced resistance to disease in crop plants by manipulation of the regulatory networks underlying expression of inducible defense responses.

ACKNOWLEDGMENTS

We thank Valerie Zatorski for preparation of the manuscript. This research was supported by grants to C.J.L. from the Samuel Roberts Nobel Foundation and the USDA. S.D.C. is a NSF Plant Biology Fellow, M.D. is a NATO–CNRS Fellow. R.A.D. thanks the Royal Society for a travel grant.

REFERENCES

Cramer, C.L., T.B. Ryder, J.N. Bell and C.J. Lamb. 1985. Rapid switching of plant gene expression by fungal elicitor. *Science* **227**: 1240.

Dangl, J.L., K.D. Hauffe, S. Lipphardt, K. Hahlbrock, and D. Scheel. 1987. Parsley protoplasts retain differential responsiveness to u.v. light and fungal elicitor. *EMBO J.* **6**: 2551.

Lamb, C.J., J.N. Bell, D.R. Corbin, M.A. Lawton, M.C. Mehdy, T.B. Ryder, N. Sauer, and M.H. Walter. 1987. Activation of defense genes in response to elicitor and infection. In *Molecular strategies for crop protection* (ed. C. Arntzen and C.A. Ryan), p. 49. Alan R. Liss, New York.

Lawton, M.A. and C.J. Lamb. 1987. Transcriptional activation of plant defense genes by fungal elicitor, wounding and infection. *Mol. Cell. Biol.* **7**: 335.

Ryder, T.B., S.A. Hedrick, J.N. Bell, X. Liang, S.D. Clouse, and C.J. Lamb. 1987. Organization and differential activation of a gene family encoding the plant defense enzyme chalcone synthase in *Phaseolus vulgaris. Mol. Gen. Genet.* **210**: 219.

Walker, J.C., E.A. Howard, E.S. Dennis, and W.J. Peacock. 1987. DNA sequences required for anaerobic expression of the maize alcohol dehydrogenase 1 gene. *Proc. Natl. Acad. Sci.* **84**: 6624.

Expression in Plants of a Bromoxynil-specific Bacterial Nitrilase That Confers Herbicide Resistance

D.M. Stalker, K.E. McBride, and L.D. Malyi

Calgene, Inc., Davis, California 95616

Bacterial isolates have been identified in bromoxynil (3,5-dibromo-4-hydroxybenzonitrile)-contaminated soil samples via bromoxynil enrichment cultures. A number of pure isolates have been shown to degrade this herbicide efficiently. Characterization of the major metabolite species from each bromoxynil-degrading organism has identifed the compound 3,5-dibromo-4-hydroxybenzoic acid, indicating the presence of a bromoxynil-specific nitrilase. One such organism has been identified as *Klebsiella pneumoniae* subspecies *ozaenae*. A plasmid-encoded gene, 1.2 kb in size, has been cloned in *Escherichia coli* and encodes a polypeptide with a molecular weight of 38,000. The bromoxynil-specific nitrilase gene (*bxn*) has been utilized to construct chimeric genes for expression in plants. Expression of the bacterial enzyme in transgenic tomato plants resulted in high levels of resistance of these plants to commercial applications of bromoxynil.

Both microbial populations and tolerant plants can transform the cyano group of nitrilic herbicides. Soil perfusion studies have shown that the cyano group on bromoxynil degradation by a *Flexibacterium* sp. (Collins 1973; Smith and Cullimore 1974) revealed the presence of the amide and acid products of the herbicide, and a corresponding study in wheat demonstrated that the cyano group is hydrolyzed to the corresponding amide and carboxylic acid products (Buckland et al. 1973). These observations suggest that the cyano moiety of the molecule is important for its toxic properties to microorganisms and plants and that removal of this constituent would essentially detoxify the compound.

Recently, a soil bacterium, *K. ozaenae*, was isolated that utilizes bromoxynil as a sole nitrogen source and encodes a nitrilase rapidly converting bromoxynil to its metabolite 3,5-

dibromo-4-hydroxybenzoic acid (McBride et al. 1986). The enzyme exhibits high specificity for bromoxynil as substrate. The gene (*bxn*) encoding a bromoxynil-specific nitrilase is plasmid encoded in *K. ozaenae* (Stalker et al. 1987). The *bxn* gene has subsequently been cloned as a 1.2-kb *PstI-HincII* DNA segment that expresses a 38,000-molecular-weight polypeptide in *E. coli* (Stalker et al. 1988).

Construction of a Chimeric Gene for Plant Transformation and Expression in Transgenic Plants

The *bxn* gene, encoding the bromoxynil-specific nitrilase, has been inserted into the plant expression cassette pCGN46, which contains the constitutive mannopine synthase (*mas*) promoter and octopine synthase (*ocs*) 3' region (Comai et al. 1985). This chimeric gene (*mas/bxn/ocs*) was cloned into the disarmed binary vector plasmid pCGN783, which contains border sequences and the cauliflower mosaic virus (CaMV) 35S promoter/*nptII* gene cassette as a selectable marker for plant transformation. The resulting plasmid (pBrx29) was introduced in disarmed *Agrobacterium tumefaciens* strains and cocultivated with tomato explants (Fillatti et al. 1987).

Of the 70 original nitrilase-positive independent kanamycin-resistant transformants (T1 plants) generated by transforming plants with *A. tumefaciens* containing pBrx29, five independent events have been open-pollinated after initial screening by spraying 1.0 pound active ingredient (ai)/acre of BUCTRIL (commercial formulation of bromoxynil). The T2-derived progeny were subjected to genetic analysis by spraying 200 plants from each transformation event with 0.5 pounds ai/acre BUCTRIL for genetic analysis and to maximum dose rate by spraying 300 progeny with BUCTRIL from 0.5 to 4.0 pounds ai/acre.

CONCLUSIONS

1. High-level resistance (8- to 16-fold) can be obtained by constitutively expressing the bromoxynil-specific nitrilase in transgenic plants. Normal field application rates are 0.25–0.5 pound ai/acre.
2. The trait is inheritable and stable.
3. Even though the biochemical target of bromoxynil is localized within the chloroplast, high-level resistance in tomato

has been achieved by expression of the enzyme in the cell cytoplasm. Chloroplast targeting is not required.

4. Resistance phenotype is somewhat related to nitrilase levels in the individual transformant. If the event is expressing enzyme at reasonable levels, the resistant phenotype is not readily distinguishable between heterozygous and homozygous plants in the T2 progeny spray experiments.

5. Expression of nitrilase at high levels does not appear to harm plant growth or development. Production of the metabolite (3,5-dibromo-4-hydroxybenzoate) at presumed high level does not appear to inhibit plant growth or development.

REFERENCES

Buckland, J., R.E. Collins, and E.M. Pullin. 1973. Metabolism of bromoxynil octanoate in growing wheat. *Pestic. Sci.* **4:** 149.

Collins, R.F. 1973. Perfusion studies with bromoxynil octanoate in soil. *Pestic. Sci.* **4:** 181.

Comai, L., D. Facciotti, W.R. Hiatt, G. Thompson, R.E. Rose, and D.M. Stalker. 1985. Expression in plants of a mutant *aroA* gene from *Salmonella typhimurium* confers tolerance to glyphosate. *Nature* **317:** 741.

Fillatti, J.J., J. Kiser, B. Rose, and L. Comai. 1987. Efficient transformation of tomato and the introduction and expression of a gene for herbicide resistance. *Tomato Biotech.* p. 199.

McBride, K.E., J.W. Kenny, and D.M. Stalker. 1986. Metabolism of the herbicide bromoxynil by *Klebsiella pneumoniae* subsp. *ozaenae*. *Appli. Environ. Microbiol.* **52:** 325.

Smith, A.E. and D.R. Cullimore. 1974. The *in vitro* degradation of the herbicide bromoxynil. *Can. J. Microbiol.* **20:** 773.

Stalker, D.M. and K.E. McBride. 1987. Cloning and expression in *E. coli* of a *Klebsiella ozaenae* plasmid-borne gene encoding a nitrilase specific for the herbicide bromoxynil. *J. Bacteriol.* **169:** 955.

Stalker, D.M., L.D. Malyi, and K.E. McBride. 1988. Purification and properties of a nitrilase specific for the herbicide bromoxynil and corresponding nucleotide sequence analysis of the *bxn* gene. *J. Biol. Chem.* (in press).

Stable and Heritable Inhibition of the Expression of Nopaline Synthase in Tobacco Expressing Antisense RNA

S.J. Rothstein, J. DiMaio, M. Strand, and D. Rice

CIBA-GEIGY Corporation, Research Triangle Park
North Carolina 27709

Antisense RNA was originally found as a naturally occurring mechanism to control gene expression in bacteria (Simons and Kleckner 1983; Mizuno et al. 1984). Its synthesis has been shown to decrease the level of gene expression in a variety of organisms besides bacteria, including *Dictyostelium* (Crowley et al. 1985), *Drosophila* (Rosenberg et al. 1985), and mammalian cells (Kim and Wold 1985). It has been demonstrated that it is possible to inhibit gene expression in transient expression experiments in *Xenopus* oocytes (Melton 1985), mammalian cells (Izant and Weintraub 1984), and carrot protoplasts (Ecker and Davis 1986). The isolation of many types of mutants in plants is still difficult, and it has not yet proved possible to construct defined mutations by gene replacement via homologous recombination. Therefore, although it is relatively straightforward to increase the expression of an isolated gene, it is at present much more difficult to decrease its expression. In those cases where the construction of a useful cultivar or tissue culture line requires a decrease in the synthesis of a particular gene product, the expression of antisense RNA could be very useful.

The mechanism by which antisense RNA inhibits expression of a gene has been shown to vary, depending on the system studied. It can inhibit translation presumably by preventing ribosome binding (Simons and Kleckner 1983; Izant and Weintraub 1984; Mizuno et al. 1984), it can prevent the mRNA from being transported from the nucleus through the formation of double-stranded RNA (Kim and Wold 1985), or it can cause increased degradation of the mRNA (Crowley et al. 1985) through the formation of double-stranded RNA. The efficacy of the antisense RNA appears to depend upon the mechanism of inhibition. For example, a large excess of antisense RNA was required to achieve a meaningful inhibition of expression when it prevented transport from the nucleus (Kim and Wold 1985). In contrast, where degradation of double-stranded RNA was shown to be the presumptive mechanism (Crowley et al. 1985), the antisense RNA did not have to be present in excess.

Construction of a Nopaline Synthase Antisense Gene and Transformation of Tobacco

The wild-type nopaline synthase (*nos*) gene had been trans-formed previously into the tobacco cultivar SR1 (de Framond et al. 1986). This original transformant was self-pollinated, and seedlings were tested for *nos* activity. One of these progeny, designated T2-16, was used in this study. A *nos* antisense gene was constructed by first inserting a restriction site 10 bp up-stream of the transcription initiation site via in vitro muta-genesis. Approximately the first two thirds of the *nos* gene can be isolated using this new restriction site and an internal *Bam*HI site. The fragment was inserted into the cauliflower mosaic virus (CaMV) 35S promoter cassette pCIB710 (Roth-stein et al. 1987) in the correct orientation for the expression of antisense RNA. This antisense-expressing gene was then in-serted into the plant-transformation vector pCIB743 (Rothstein et al. 1987) to make pCIB749. pCIB749 was used to transform T2-16 plants by the leaf-disk transformation method (Horsch et al. 1985), using hygromycin resistance as the plant-selectable marker. Control plants were transformed with the vector pCIB743. Hygromycin-resistant seedlings were grown in agar in GA-7 containers prior to being potted in soil and transferred to the greenhouse.

nos Activity in the Transformed Plants

The transformed plants were analyzed for *nos* activity. When analyzing the control plants transformed with the vector alone, it became obvious that the amount of enzyme activity varied depending on the tissue used. This variability was found to depend on the developmental stage of the tissue and the age of the plant. It was therefore essential to analyze tissue of very similar developmental stages when comparing different trans-formed plants. There was still some variability in the control plants due to the difficulties in having all the initial trans-formed plants at exactly the same developmental stage. Even so, the plants transformed with the *nos* antisense gene had considerably lower enzyme activity than the control plants. This decrease in average enzyme activity varied from 8- to 50-fold, depending on the leaf tissue analyzed. In older greenhouse-grown plants, the decrease in activity was less than that in the younger plants grown in GA-7 jars in vitro.

Steady-state *nos* mRNA Levels Are Decreased by the Antisense RNA

To analyze the steady-state levels of sense and antisense transcripts in the transformed plants, total leaf RNA was analyzed via RNase protection experiments (Zinn et al. 1983). The level of mRNA was found to be decreased considerably (~8- to 10-fold) in the plants transformed with the *nos* antisense gene. A similar result was found when the mRNA was analyzed by RNA transfer blots, although quantitation was not possible due to the low intensity of the signal for the plants expressing antisense RNA. However, the *nos* mRNA for control plants could be detected, with the amount of mRNA present being approximately the same for different control plants. Therefore, it appears as though the primary mechanism by which the antisense RNA inhibits *nos* expression is through a decrease in mRNA level. Steady-state levels of the antisense RNA in the plant samples were determined in the same fashion. The levels of antisense RNA found in plants transformed with pCIB749 are approximately tenfold higher than the amount of *nos* mRNA. However, this level of antisense RNA is approximately the same as the *nos* mRNA levels found in control plants (transformed with pCIB743). Therefore, the antisense RNA does not have to be present in great excess in order to achieve a significant reduction in expression.

Cosegregation of the Decrease in *nos* Expression with the Antisense Gene in Progeny Plants

A genetic analysis of the transformed plants was performed to demonstrate heritability of the antisense gene and phenotype. The pCIB749-transformed plants, which were *nos*+/antisense+, were crossed to wild-type (*nos*−) tobacco. The T2-16 line originally transformed was heterozygous for the *nos* gene. If transformants were also heterozygous for the antisense gene, one would expect a progeny ratio of 1 *nos*+/antisense+:1 *nos*+/antisense−:1 *nos*−/antisense+:1 *nos*−/antisense−. Two of the pCIB749-transformed plants were crossed with the Coker 176 line of tobacco. Sixteen progeny plants were tested for nopaline production and hygromycin resistance. (Because hygromycin resistance was adjacent to the antisense gene on the DNA transferred to the plants, it should be very closely linked to that gene.) For nopaline determinations, a soluble extract was made from leaf tissue from each of these plants and equalized with respect to protein concentration. After paper electrophoresis, the samples were stained for the presence of nopaline. The results (see Fig. 1) for the *nos⁺*/hygromycin-resistant and

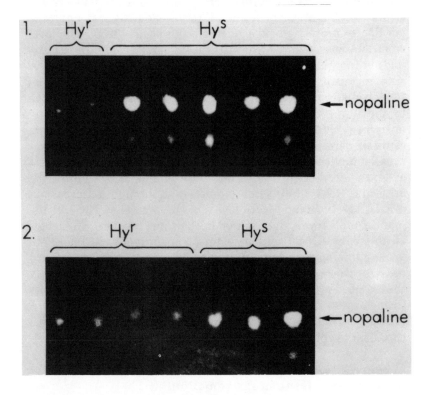

Figure 1 Nopaline present in progeny plants. pCIB749-transformed T2-16 plants were backcrossed to wild-type tobacco. Sixteen progeny plants from each cross were tested for hygromycin resistance (Hyʳ) and for the presence of nopaline. Hygromycin-resistant plants should contain the *nos* antisense RNA-expressing gene, whereas hygromycin-sensitive (Hyˢ) plants should not. Those plants that did not make nopaline were removed from the screen. The leaf material was homogenized and each sample was equalized for its protein concentration. The samples were analyzed by paper electrophoresis and stained for the presence of nopaline. Two sets of progeny plants are shown.

nos+/hygromycin-sensitive plants demonstrate a clear linkage between hygromycin resistance and a decreased level of nopaline in the progeny. Therefore, not only is the expression of antisense RNA effective in reducing the expression of the *nos* gene, but this effect is stably inherited.

CONCLUSIONS

The inhibition of expression of the *nos* gene by antisense RNA demonstrates that it is possible to use this technology to alter phenotype at the whole-plant level. Not only is this inhibition maintained throughout the life of the plant, but it is stably inherited in progeny plants. It appears that the primary means by which the antisense RNA inhibits expression is through a decrease in the level of the mRNA. We propose the mechanism to be the formation of double-stranded RNA, which is degraded more rapidly than free mRNA. It is possible that other mechanisms, such as decreased translation of the mRNA, are also important contributors to reduced gene expression. Although there will likely be important differences in the efficacy of using antisense RNA to inhibit the expression of other genes in plants, the ability to decrease expression of the *nos* gene demonstrates the potential feasibility of this approach.

REFERENCES

Crowley, T.E., W. Nellen, R.H. Gomer, and R.A. Firtel. 1985. Phenocopy of discoidin I-mutants by antisense transformation in *Dictyostelium*. *Cell* **43**: 633.

de Framond, A.J., E.W. Back, W.S. Chilton, L. Kayes, and M.-D. Chilton. 1986. Two unlinked T-DNAs can transform the same tobacco plant cell and segregate in the F1 generation. *Mol. Gen. Genet.* **202**: 125.

Ecker, J.R. and R.W. Davis. 1986. Inhibition of gene expression in plant cells by expression of antisense RNA. *Proc. Natl. Acad. Sci.* **83**: 5372.

Horsch, R.B., J.E. Fry, N.L. Hoffmann, P. Eichholtz, S.G. Rogers, and R.T. Fraley. 1985. A simple and general method for transferring genes into plants. *Science* **227**: 1229.

Izant, J.G. and H. Weintraub. 1984. Inhibition of thymidine kinase gene expression by anti-sense RNA: A molecular approach to genetic analysis. *Cell* **36**: 1007.

Kim, S.K. and B.J. Wold. 1985. Stable reduction of thymidine kinase activity in cells expressing high levels of anti-sense RNA. *Cell* **42**: 129.

Melton, D.A. 1985. Injected anti-sense RNAs specifically block messenger RNA translation in vivo. *Proc. Natl. Acad. Sci.* **82**: 144.

Mizuno, T., M. Chou, and M. Inouye. 1984. A unique mechanism regulating gene expression: Translational inhibition by a complementary RNA transcript (mic RNA). *Proc. Natl. Acad. Sci.* **81:** 1966.

Rosenberg, G.B., A. Preiss, E. Seifert, H. Jackle, and D.C. Knipple. 1985. Production of phenocopies by Kruppel antisense RNA injection into *Drosophila* embryos. *Nature* **313:** 703.

Rothstein, S.J., K.N. Lahners, R.J. Lotstein, N.B. Carozzi, S.M. Jayne, and D.A. Rice. 1987. Promoter cassettes, antibiotic-resistance genes, and vectors for plant transformation. *Gene* **53:** 153.

Simons, R.W. and N. Kleckner. 1983. Translational control of IS10 transposition. *Cell* **34:** 683.

Zinn, K., D. DiMaio, and T. Maniatis. 1983. Identification of two distinct regulatory regions adjacent to the human-interferon gene. *Cell* **34:** 865.

Transformation to Produce Virus-resistant Plants

R.N. Beachy,[1] R.S. Nelson,[1] J. Register III,[1] R.T. Fraley,[2] and N. Tumer[2]

[1]Department of Biology, Washington University
St. Louis, Missouri 63130

[2]Monsanto Company, St. Louis, Missouri 63198

Although non-host-resistant mechanisms prevent many viruses from establishing infections in most plants, there are substantial numbers of plant viruses that cause diseases, some of which are responsible for significant crop losses. Disease symptoms can include (1) mild or severe chlorosis on infected leaves; (2) stunting due to shortened internode distances or overall dwarf stature; (3) fewer reproductive organs or reduced fertilization; and (4) production of low-quality fruit. These symptoms may be the direct or indirect result of viral infection.

Resistance to virus diseases has, until recently, been derived by incorporating "genes for resistance," generally found in wild relatives of the plant in question by the classical approaches used in plant breeding. Such an approach often requires 15 years or more to introduce the desired resistance trait and to remove unwanted genetic traits. An alternate approach has been used to protect plants from infection by preinfecting the plant with a related virus that is attenuated in disease symptoms but not replication. These preinfected plants are "cross-protected" against infection by other related strains of the protective virus. Cross-protection has been successfully applied to control several disease situations but has found limited use often because of the effort required to isolate an attenuated virus strain. There are a number of inherent problems that accompany the widespread inoculation of even a mild virus strain under agricultural situations.

Recently, we demonstrated the production of plants that are partially resistant to viral infection by using a plant-transformation approach. We describe here the results of recent experiments from several laboratories to produce resistance to a number of different viruses and the results of field and greenhouse studies with plants that are resistant to tobacco mosaic virus (TMV). These studies indicate that the

47

approach may be widely applicable to produce field-level resistance against a number of different plant viruses.

Producing Virus Resistance in Transgenic Plants

A number of different studies were carried out in the 1970s and early 1980s documenting that cross-protection against viruses and viroids could be engendered by first infecting the host with a mild strain of the pathogen. However, as reviewed by several authors (Hamilton 1980; Palukaitis and Zaitlin 1985), there was widespread disagreement about the viral gene product (or products) that is responsible for protection. The results of experiments with viroids (which encode no known protein) and defective strains of viruses (producing nonfunctional structural proteins) suggested that protection might be caused by interactions between RNA molecules during replication or translation that block or delay infection by the superinfecting virus or viroid. Equally convincing results suggested that viral capsid proteins were, in some way, responsible for the protection (Sherwood and Fulton 1982).

We set out to express different portions of the genome of TMV as chimeric nuclear genes in transgenic plants. The chimeric genes expressed either sense or antisense sequences of the viral genome, some of which encoded a known viral gene product. In early experiments, genes were driven by expression of the promoter for the 19S RNA of cauliflower mosaic virus (CaMV). However, the levels of accumulation of RNA transcripts or protein products were relatively low, and no resistance was observed (P. Powell Abel and R.N. Beachy, unpubl.). When the CaMV 35S promoter was used, however, levels of RNA and protein accumulation were substantially greater, and we were able to detect resistance in transgenic plants that accumulated specific viral gene products. A summary of the sequences of TMV-RNA that have been expressed in transgenic plants and the results of the disease resistance assays are presented in Table 1.

On the basis of these results, we suggested that the most promising approach for imparting virus resistance in transgenic plants was through expression of the capsid protein gene, and we described a general approach that could be used to isolate capsid protein sequences from any virus, cause its expression in transgenic plants, and determine the degree of virus resistance (Beachy et al. 1987). In recent months, other workers have reported that a similar approach taken with the

Table 1 TMV Sequences Expressed in Transgenic Plants and Effects on Disease Development

Nucleotides expressed	Transcript polarity sense/anti-sense	Viral cistrons encoded	Protein(s) detected	Relative disease resistance	Reference
3335–6395	sense	part of viral replicase movement protein (30 kD) capsid protein	none	n.d.	Beachy et al. (1987b)
3336–6395	antisense	—	none	n.d.	Beachy et al. (1987b)
4855–5868	sense	30-kD movement protein	movement protein	n.d.	Deom et al. (1987)
5707–6395	sense	capsid protein	capsid protein	++++	Powell Abel et al. (1986)
5705–6395	antisense	—	none	+	P. Powell Abel et al. (in prep.)

+ indicates a relatively low degree of disease resistance; ++++ indicates a substantially higher level of disease resistance; n.d. indicates not detected.

49

capsid protein gene of alfalfa mosaic virus (AlMV) successfully conferred resistance to AlMV in transgenic tobacco and tomato plants (Loesch-Fries et al. 1987; Tumer et al. 1987; Van Dun et al. 1987). Other workers recently found that by using a similar approach resistance was achieved against potato virus X (Hemenway et al. 1988) and cucumber mosaic virus (Cuozzo et al. 1988). Each of these viruses has morphological characteristics different from those of TMV, and because of this and other reasons, it is anticipated that resistance can be produced against viruses in a number of different groups, presumably in a number of different plant species.

Characterizing Virus Resistance in Transgenic Plants

The resistance in transgenic plants that express viral capsid proteins has the following characteristics:

1. In the case of TMV and AlMV, resistance is greater against virus than against viral RNA (Loesch-Fries et al. 1987; Nelson et al. 1987).

2. The degree of resistance is positively correlated with the level of gene expression (G. Clark et al., in prep.). To confer resistance against TMV, transgenic plants that accumulate capsid protein to less than 0.005% (w/w) of cell protein are less tolerant to infection than those that accumulate 0.05% capsid protein.

3. Transgenic plants that accumulate capsid protein have 70–95% fewer sites of successful infection following inoculation with virus than plants that do not accumulate capsid protein (Loesch-Fries et al. 1987; Nelson et al. 1987; Tumer et al. 1987; Van Dun et al. 1987). Resistance is also expressed in protoplasts isolated from transgenic plants (Loesch-Fries et al. 1986; J. Register and R.N. Beachy, in prep.) and is reflected in reduced numbers of infected protoplasts.

4. Capsid protein-expressing plants whose inoculated leaves become infected have significantly lower rates of systemic disease development than nontransgenic plants (Powell Abel et al. 1986; Tumer et al. 1987).

5. Resistance against TMV results from accumulation of capsid protein per se, rather than capsid protein mRNA (P. Powell Abel et al., in prep.).

6. Plants that accumulate capsid protein of the U_1 strain of TMV are protected against a variety of strains of TMV and tomato mosaic virus (Nelson et al. 1988).

7. Resistance against viruses not related to the virus from which the capsid protein gene was taken is considerably less (<1/1000) than that against related viruses (E. Anderson et al., in prep.). No resistance was recorded against *Pseudomonas syringa* pv *pisi*, which causes localized necrosis in tobacco plants.

MECHANISMS PROPOSED

Studies designed to elucidate the mechanism(s) of the protection in engineered plants must accommodate most or all of the observations described above. Recent unpublished data from our research group implicate a role of the capsid protein, rather than its mRNA, in protection against infection by TMV (P. Powell Abel et al., unpubl.). Because the capsid protein is the active moiety, its function could be (1) to induce a host response that causes a specific (rather than broad) resistance to viruses closely related to that from which the capsid protein gene was taken; (2) to reincapsidate partially or fully stripped viral RNA, thereby blocking expression of the challenge virus; (3) to block an initial step in the infection process that causes the release of the viral RNA; (4) any combination of the above. Because of the results of experiments showing that infection with TMV-RNA (Nelson et al. 1987) or with TMV particles treated at elevated pH (J. Register and R.N. Beachy, in prep.) largely overcomes the protection, we favor a model that includes a blockage in an uncoating step early in the infection process. However, there may be additional mechanisms at work that account for the reduced rate of systemic movement in transgenic plants *if* infection occurs on the inoculated leaves (Powell Abel et al. 1986; L. Wisniewski and R.N. Beachy, unpubl.).

RESISTANCE UNDER FIELD CONDITIONS

Following extensive experimentation under glasshouse and growth-chamber conditions, permission was granted to conduct a test under field conditions (conducted in collaboration with Dr. X. Delannay, Monsanto Company). The data recently collected and compiled documented that resistance was as great or greater in the field experiment than in glasshouse trials. In these trials, less than 10% of the capsid-protein-expressing plants developed symptoms of viral infection. Likewise, these plants accumulated much less virus than plants that did not express the capsid protein gene. The yields of tomatoes on transgenic plants were unaffected by inoculation with TMV, and equivalent to the yields of the control (nontransgenic) plants that were not infected. As expected, noninfected control plants suffered a yield loss of 25–34% due to the infection by the U_1-strain (Nelson et al. 1988).

Although further field tests are needed to demonstrate the application of genetically engineered cross-protection against other viruses, the results of these first trials indicate that this approach will be useful to confer protection against viral infections under standard agronomic situations.

REFERENCES

Beachy, R.N., S.G. Rogers, and R.T. Fraley. 1987a. Genetic transformation to confer resistance to plant virus disease. In *Genetic engineering* (ed. J.K. Setlow), vol. 9, p. 224. Plenum Publishing, New York.

Beachy, R.N., D.M. Stark, C.M. Deom, M.J. Oliver, and R.T. Fraley. 1987b. Expression of sequences of tobacco mosaic virus in transgenic plants and their role in disease resistance. In *Tailoring genes for crop improvement* (ed. G. Bruening et al.) p. 169. Plenum Press, New York.

Cuozzo, M., K.M. O'Connell, W. Kaniewski, R.-X. Fang, N.-H. Chua, and N.E. Tumer. 1988. Viral protection in transgenic plants expressing the cucumber mosaic virus coat protein or its antisense RNA. *Bio/Technology* (in press).

Deom, C.M., M.J. Oliver, and R.N. Beachy. 1987. The 30-kilodalton gene product of tobacco mosaic virus potentiates virus movement. *Science* **237**: 389.

Hamilton, R.I. 1980. Defenses triggered by previous invaders: Viruses. In *Plant disease: An advanced treatise* (ed. I.G. Horsfall and E.B. Cowling), vol. 5, p. 279. Academic Press, New York.

Hemenway, C., R.-X. Fang, W.K. Kaniewski, N.-H. Chua, and N.E. Tumer. 1988. Analysis of the mechanism of protection in transgenic plants expressing the potato virus X coat protein or its antisense RNA. *EMBO J.* (in press).

Loesch-Fries, L.S., E. Halk, D. Merlo, N. Jarvis, S. Nelson, K. Krahn, and L. Burhop. 1986. Expression of alfalfa mosaic virus coat protein and anti-sense cDNA in transformed tobacco tissue. In *Molecular strategies for crop protection* (ed. D.J. Arntzen and C. Ryan), p. 221. Alan R. Liss, New York.

Loesch-Fries, L.S., D. Merlo, T. Zinnen, L. Burhop, K. Hill, K. Krahn, N. Jarvis, S. Nelson, and E. Halk. 1987. Expression of alfalfa mosaic virus RNA 4 in trangenic plants confers virus resistance. *EMBO J.* **6**: 1845.

Nelson, R.S., P. Powell Abel, and R.N. Beachy. 1987. Lesions and virus accumulation in inoculated transgenic tobacco plants expressing the coat protein gene of tobacco mosaic virus. *Virology* **158**: 126.

Nelson, R.S., S.M. McCormick, X. Delannay, P. Dubé, J. Layton, E.J. Anderson, M. Kaniewska, R.K. Proksch, R.B. Horsch, S.G. Rogers, R.T. Fraley, and R.N. Beachy. 1988. Virus tolerance, plant growth, and field performance of transgenic tomato plants expressing coat protein from tobacco mosaic virus. *Bio/Technology* (in press).

Palukaitis, P. and M. Zaitlin. 1985. A model to explain the "cross-protection" phenomenon shown by plant viruses and viroids. In *Plant-microbe interactions* (ed. T. Kosuge and E. Nester), vol. 1, p. 42. MacMillan Publishing, New York.

Powell Abel, P., R.S. Nelson, B. De, N. Hoffmann, S.G. Rogers, R.T. Fraley, and R.N. Beachy. 1986. Delay of disease development in transgenic plants that express the tobacco mosaic virus coat protein gene. *Science* **232**: 738.

Sherwood, J.L. and R.W. Fulton., 1982. The specific involvement of coat protein in tobacco mosaic virus cross protection. *Virology* **119**: 150.

Tumer, N.E., K.M. O'Connell, R.S. Nelson, P.R. Sanders, R.N. Beachy, R.T. Fraley, and D.M. Shah. 1987. Expression of alfalfa mosaic virus coat protein gene confers cross-protection in transgenic tobacco and tomato plants. *EMBO J.* **6**: 1181.

Van Dun, C.M.P., J.F. Bol, and L. Van Vloten-Doting. 1987. Expression of alfalfa mosaic virus and tobacco rattle virus coat protein genes in transgenic tobacco plants. *Virology* **159**: 299.

Creation and Field Testing of Sulfonylurea-resistant Crops

S. Knowlton, B.J. Mazur, and C.J. Arntzen

Agricultural Biotechnology Division, Experimental Station
E.I. du Pont de Nemours and Company
Wilmington, Delaware 19898

The sulfonylureas are a relatively large family of very potent herbicides that have extremely low mammalian toxicity. A vast number of structurally related compounds have been synthesized and identified as herbicidally active. Many can be used to control a broad spectrum of weeds, whereas others are selective in their ability to kill weeds without causing injury to target crops. Soil residual properties also vary. Typically, sulfonylureas may be applied at rates of a few grams per hectare, in contrast to some older classes of herbicides that require use rates of several pounds per hectare to achieve effective weed control. These characteristics, coupled with an understanding of the mode of action of these compounds, have made engineering sulfonylurea-resistant crop plants an attractive area for commercial development.

The sulfonylureas act by inhibiting acetolactate synthase (ALS), the first common enzyme in the biosynthetic pathways of the branched chain amino acids leucine, isoleucine, and valine. Their mode of action was first discovered in a microbial system, in which bacteria were shown to be sensitive to sulfonylureas when grown on minimal media but resistant when the media were supplemented with branched chain amino acids (LaRossa and Schloss 1984). Biochemical and genetic studies on the enzyme confirmed ALS as the molecular target. Subsequent experiments established that ALS was also the target in both yeast (Falco and Dumas 1985) and plants (Chaleff and Mauvais 1984; Ray 1984).

ALS is also inhibited by a number of structurally unrelated herbicidal compounds, which include the imidazolinones (Shaner et al. 1984), the active ingredient in several American Cyanamid herbicides, and the triazolopyrimidines (T.R. Hawkes et al., in prep.) developed by Dow. LaRossa et al. (1987) have proposed that ALS inactivation results in particularly potent herbicidal activity, both because branched chain amino acids are depleted and because the ALS substrate α-ketobutyrate accumulates and is toxic to the cells.

Engineering resistance to herbicides has been accomplished using several strategies. Because plants and microbes which are naturally tolerant to herbicides possess mechanisms for detoxification (Sweetser et al. 1982), tolerance can be achieved by cloning and introducing into plants genes that encode proteins that inactivate these compounds metabolically. De Block et al. (1987) created herbicide-resistant plants by expressing a bacterial enzyme that detoxifies phosphinothricin. Alternatively, Shah et al. (1986) have demonstrated that overproduction of a sensitive target enzyme in transgenic plants can result in herbicide tolerance. Overexpression of 5-enol-pyruvylshikimate-3 phosphate synthase conferred tolerance to glyphosate in petunia. Resistance can also be achieved by introducing into plants a gene encoding a form of the target enzyme that is insensitive to the inhibitors. The following material will focus on this latter approach to engineer sulfonylurea resistance in crop plants.

Cloning and Characterization of Plant ALS Genes

The use of microbes as models for higher plants allowed the cloning and sequencing of an ALS gene from yeast (Falco and Dumas 1985; Falco et al. 1985). A high level of homology between the cloned yeast ALS gene and a bacterial ALS gene suggested that higher plant ALS genes could be identified by heterologous hybridizations. The yeast ALS gene was used to probe genomic libraries from the higher plants *Arabidopsis* and tobacco. Phage carrying putative ALS genes from both species were isolated (Mazur et al. 1985). The genes from tobacco and *Arabidopsis* were subsequently mapped and sequenced, and their deduced amino acid sequences were determined (Mazur et al. 1987).

The two genes encode proteins of 667 (tobacco) and 670 (*Arabidopsis*) amino acids, with predicted molecular weights of approximately 73,000. Neither gene has introns. Except for the 5′ end of the coding sequences, presumed to encode the chloroplast transit sequences, the two genes are highly conserved. This suggests that ALS genes from one plant species are likely to be functional when introduced into heterologous species. The cloned *Arabidopsis* and tobacco ALS genes have been used as hybridization probes to isolate ALS genes from sulfonylurea-resistant lines of tobacco (K.Y. Lee et al., in prep.) and *Arabidopsis* (Haughn et al. 1987).

Cloning and Introduction of Sulfonylurea-resistant ALS Genes in Plants

Tobacco lines resistant to sulfonylurea herbicides were first produced by Chaleff and Ray (1984), using cell-culture methods. Genetic analysis indicated that the mutations segregated as single semidominant mutations in two linkage groups, designated C3 and S4. The S4 line was subjected to further selection on increased levels of the herbicide. From these experiments, a highly resistant line, able to tolerate levels of herbicide 1000-fold greater than wild-type tissue, was identified (Chaleff et al. 1987). This line was designated Hra. The Hra mutation was shown to be genetically linked to the original S4 mutation. All three mutant tobacco lines had a form of ALS that was less sensitive to sulfonylurea herbicides than the wild-type enzyme was. The sensitive tobacco ALS gene, which had been cloned previously, was used as a hybridization probe to isolate genes from C3 and Hra genomic libraries (K.Y. Lee et al., in prep.). Mutant and wild-type genes representing each locus were sequenced, and the mutations were identified. Whereas the C3 mutation results in a change of a single amino acid, the highly resistant Hra phenotype results from two amino acid substitutions in ALS.

The Hra gene has been used to transform cells from a number of heterologous plant species to sulfonylurea resistance, including tomato, sugarbeet, rape, lettuce, alfalfa, and melon. The most extensive experiments, including field trials, have been done with commercial varieties of tobacco in a collaborative agreement with Northrup King, Inc.

Sixty-six stably transformed lines of five Northrup King tobacco cultivars have been characterized in biochemical, molecular, and genetic experiments. The relative proportions of resistant to sensitive ALS activity in leaf extracts from each primary transformant have been determined. The proportions vary, ranging broadly from 30% to 70% resistant activity in the presence of 10 parts per billion (ppb) of a sulfonylurea compound. Segregation of the resistant phenotype in the progeny of self-fertilized transformants has also been examined. The majority of these lines have insertions at a single genetic locus. Several lines have multiple, genetically unlinked ALS gene insertions. In some cases, high levels of resistant enzyme activity can be correlated with the number of gene integrations. In other cases, the high level of resistant enzyme activity presumably results from position effects unique to the insertion event. Six lines, chosen as a result of these experiments, were tested in field experiments at the Northrup King tobacco breeding farm in Laurinburg, North Carolina.

Field Tests

The field tests were designed to determine the efficacy of the Hra gene in conferring sulfonylurea resistance under actual growing conditions. For this reason, the test location was chosen, in part, on the basis of the weeds predominant in that field. The plots were sprayed with 1x, 2x, and 4x field application rates of a sulfonylurea herbicide. After 14 days, the plots were rated and photographed (Fig. 1). Whereas wild-type control plants showed severe damage (arrested growth, yellow and necrotic leaves), the transformed lines appeared completely unharmed even at the highest rates tested. The plots were rated several more times during the growing season. No subsequent herbicide applications were required because the weeds were effectively controlled by the initial treatment. With time, non-

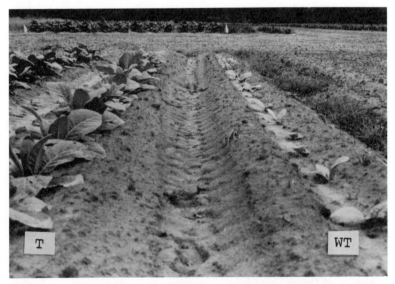

Figure 1 Field test of sulfonylurea-resistant transgenic tobacco. (*Foreground*) Plants transformed with the Hra gene (T) and wild-type plants (WT) were sprayed with 4x field rate of sulfonylurea.

transformed plants began to recover, and new growth was initiated. However, at no point did the nontransformed plants match the growth and vigor of the transformed lines.

The success of these experiments demonstrates that the Hra gene is able to confer useful levels of herbicide resistance in transgenic plants grown under field conditions. The ability to introduce this resistance into heterologous species should provide many exciting opportunities. New crop/gene/herbicide combinations could augment herbicide use strategies and provide greater flexibility for the farmer. Public health concerns should also be assuaged, as the sulfonylureas have proven to be nontoxic to mammals and environmentally safe, and their broader use will reduce the reliance on older compounds that have greater environmental risks.

ACKNOWLEDGMENTS
We appreciate the contributions of many of our colleagues at du Pont who have participated directly or indirectly in this work. Special thanks to Chris Kostow for plant transformations and enzyme assays, Perry Caimi for molecular analysis of transformants, Gary Fader for greenhouse spray tests, Louis Rodrigue (du Pont) and Bill Earley and Luis Lazo-Anaya (Northrup King) for field studies, and Tom Ray and Jim Yager for field plot design. The work of Julie Smith, Carl Falco, Roy Chaleff, Gary Creason, Jeff Mauvais, Chok-Fun Chui, Sharon Martin, Ray McDevitt, Mary Hartnett, Tony Guida, and Tim Ward of du Pont and Kathy Lee, Jeff Townsend, Pamela Dunsmuir, and John Bedbrook at Advanced Genetic Sciences has provided the foundation for these experiments.

REFERENCES
Chaleff, R.S. and C.J. Mauvais. 1984. Acetolactate synthase is the site of action of two sulfonylurea herbicides in higher plants. *Science* **224**: 1443.
Chaleff, R.S. and T.B. Ray. 1984. Herbicide-resistant mutants from tobacco cell cultures. *Science* **223**: 1148.
Chaleff, R.S., S.A. Sebastian, G.L. Creason, B.J. Mazur, S.C. Falco, T.B. Ray, C.J. Mauvais, and N.S. Yadav. 1987. Developing plant varieties resistant to sulfonylurea herbicides. In *Molecular strategies for crop protection* (ed. C.J. Arntzen and C.A. Ryan). Alan R. Liss, New York.
De Block, M., J. Botterman, M. Vandewiele, J. Dockx, C. Thoen, V. Gossele, N. Rao Movva, C. Thompson, M. Van Montagu, and J. Leemans. 1987. Engineering herbicide resistance in plants by expression of a detoxifying enzyme. *EMBO J.* **6**: 2513.
Falco, S.C. and K.D. Dumas. 1985. Genetic analysis of mutants of

Saccharomyces cerevisiae resistant to the herbicide sulfometuron methyl. *Genetics* **109:** 21.

Falco, S.C., K.D. Dumas, and K.J. Livak. 1985. Nucleotide sequence of the yeast *ILV2* gene which encodes acetolactate synthase. *Nucleic Acids Res.* **13:** 4011.

Haughn, G., J.K. Smith, B.J. Mazur, and C. Somerville. 1988. An *Arabidopsis* acetolactate synthase gene in tobacco confers resistance to sulfonylurea herbicides. *Mol. Gen. Genet.* (in press).

LaRossa, R.A. and J.V. Schloss. 1984. The sulfonylurea herbicide sulfometuron methyl is an extremely potent and selective inhibitor of acetolactate synthase in *Salmonella typhimurium*. *J. Biol. Chem.* **259:** 8753.

LaRossa, R.A., S.C. Falco, B.J. Mazur, K.J. Livak, J.V. Schloss, D.R. Smulski, T.K. Van Dyk, and N.S. Yadav. 1987. Microbiological identification and characterization of an amino acid biosynthetic enzyme as the site of sulfonylurea herbicide action. In *Biotechnology in agricultural chemistry* (ed. H.M. LeBaron et al.), p. 1372. American Chemical Society, Washington, D.C.

Mazur, B.J., C.-F. Chui, and J.K. Smith. 1987. Isolation and characterization of plant genes coding for acetolactate synthase, the target enzyme for two classes of herbicides. *Plant Physiol.* **85:** 1110.

Mazur, B.J., C.-F. Chui, S.C. Falco, C.J. Mauvais, and R.S. Chaleff. 1985. Cloning herbicide resistance genes into and out of plants. In *The World Biotech Report 1985*, p. 97. Online International, New York.

Ray, T.B. 1984. Site of action of chlorsulfuron. *Plant Physiol.* **75:** 827.

Shah, D.M., R.B. Horsch, H.J. Klee, G.M. Kishore, J.A. Winter, N.E. Tumer, C.M. Hironaka, P.R. Sanders, C.S. Gasser, S. Aykent, N.R. Siegel, S.G. Rogers, and R.T. Fraley. 1986. Engineering herbicide tolerance in transgenic plants. *Science* **233:** 478.

Shaner, D.L., P.C. Anderson, and M.A. Stidham. 1984. Imidazolinones (potent inhibitors of acetohydroxyacid synthase). *Plant Physiol.* **76:** 545.

Sweetser, P.B., G.S. Schow, and J.M. Hutchison. 1982. Metabolism of chlorsulfuron by plants: Biological basis for selectivity of a new herbicide for cereals. *Pestic. Biochem. Physiol.* **17:** 18.

Altering Protein and Oil-quality Traits in Seeds

S.B. Altenbach, S.S.M. Sun, and J.B. Mudd

The Plant Cell Research Institute, Inc., Dublin, California 94568

Seeds are an extremely important source of food for both man and domesticated animals. The storage materials intended for use in the germination of seeds and the early growth of seedlings, including proteins, oils, and carbohydrates, can be used to supply animals with essential amino acids, essential fatty acids, as well as calories. These storage materials can also be used for industrial purposes. Approximately 10% of vegetable oils have nonfood uses.

The use of seeds for nutrition of animals is not without problems. Cereal grains are frequently deficient in lysine, whereas the seeds of leguminous plants are frequently deficient in the sulfur-containing amino acids, cysteine and methionine. Some seeds are unsuitable for animal nutrition because of toxic components such as the glucosinolates in many seeds of cruciferous plants. Others are unsuitable because of susceptibility to autoxidation of the fatty acids, as in the case of linseed.

The goals of plant breeding in the past, present, and future and of genetic engineering in the present and future are to improve the amino acid composition of seeds in which protein is stored and to modify the oil content for either nutritional or industrial purposes. In this paper, we describe the details of our efforts to modify the amino acid composition of soybean seeds to increase the content of cysteine and methionine, and we discuss the opportunities to improve the oil composition of oil seeds.

Altering the Amino Acid Composition of Seeds

One molecular approach for altering the amino acid composition of seed proteins involves the transfer of genes that encode proteins containing large amounts of the limiting amino acid from one plant to another. For improving the quality of leguminous seed proteins that are deficient in the sulfur-containing amino acids, we have focused on a small family of proteins found in the seeds of the Brazil nut (*Bertholletia excelsa*), which are unusually rich in methionine and cysteine (Sun et al. 1987b). Our hope is that a gene encoding a sulfur-rich protein from the Brazil nut can be transferred to leguminous plants and expressed in the seeds at a level that will be sufficient to improve the overall sulfur–amino acid composition.

The sulfur-rich protein from the Brazil nut is a member of a family of small, water-soluble seed proteins that contain approximately 8% cysteine and 18% methionine. The mature protein consists of 9-kD and 3-kD subunits linked through disulfide bridges (Sun et al. 1987a). Like storage proteins from other seeds, the synthesis of the sulfur-rich protein is developmentally regulated; the protein is synthesized at a mid-maturation stage and accumulates in the mature seeds. The sulfur-rich protein is synthesized initially as a 17-kD precursor polypeptide that undergoes three proteolytic processing steps before it attains its mature form. First, a signal peptide of about 2 kD is cleaved from the precursor, leaving a 15-kD precursor that is then trimmed to a 12-kD polypeptide and finally to the 9-kD and 3-kD subunits of the sulfur-rich protein (Sun et al. 1987a).

cDNA clones representing several members of the sulfur-rich protein gene family have been isolated and sequenced (Altenbach et al. 1987). We have used one of these cDNAs to construct a chimeric gene in which the promoter region and 3' - flanking region of the phaseolin gene from French beans are linked to cDNA sequences encoding the 17-kD precursor form of the sulfur-rich protein. Using a binary vector system of *Agrobacterium tumefaciens*, we have transferred this chimeric gene to tobacco and have regenerated transformed plants.

Southern blot analysis of DNA isolated from the leaves of the transgenic tobacco plants indicates that the chimeric gene has been transferred to the tobacco plants, and analysis of RNA isolated from developing seeds indicates that the chimeric gene is transcribed. Using immunological techniques, we have found that the sulfur-rich protein is expressed in the seeds at levels that approach 5% of the total seed protein. At least some of the protein is processed to the 9-kD subunit of the mature sulfur-rich protein. However, a larger polypeptide is also found in the seeds of the transgenic plants, which probably represents one of the intermediate precursors of the sulfur-rich protein (S.B. Altenbach et al., in prep.). Currently, we are analyzing the amino acid composition of the seed proteins from the transgenic plants expressing the highest quantities of the sulfur-rich protein in hopes of determining whether the level of expression of the sulfur-rich protein in the transgenic seeds is sufficient to alter the sulfur–amino acid composition of the tobacco seeds.

Because the phaseolin–sulfur-rich protein chimeric gene appears to be expressed in the seeds of a model plant system, we are attempting to transfer the chimeric gene to several different legumes with the hope that the expression of these sequences in the seeds of leguminous plants will enhance the nutritional value of the seeds.

Altering the Oil Composition of Seeds

The goals of breeding programs and now genetic engineering laboratories in the improvement of oil quality in oil seeds can be placed in two main categories: (1) control of chain length of the fatty acids, and (2) control of the degree of unsaturation of the fatty acids.

The major drive in the control of chain length is to achieve the accumulation of 12-carbon fatty acids in the seeds of crops grown in temperate climates. The current source of 12-carbon acids (lauric acid) is coconut oil or palm kernel oil coming from the Philippines and Malaysia. The price of these materials has been subject to considerable fluctuation, so the availability of lauric acid from a crop suited to the climates of North America or Europe has considerable interest.

Control of the degree of unsaturation has been directed to the change of the oil composition of a crop like sunflower from high linoleic acid to high oleic acid. This can change the value of the oil both from the point of view of food usage and for industrial purposes because the presence of high purity oleic acid increases the possibilities for derivation at places other than the carboxyl group. Another case would be the change of a crop like linseed from high linolenic to high linoleic acid content in order to make the oil of culinary use.

In the two specific cases of control of degree of unsaturation mentioned above, sunflower and linseed, the desired goals have been reached by mutation breeding. One may ask the question whether genetic engineering could have done the job as well or better. In the case of controlling chain length, the breeding work concerns plants of the genus *Cuphea,* whereas searching for a genetic engineering solution to this problem depends on an understanding of the biochemical factors that control chain length. Very little progress has been made on this aspect of the problem.

Genetically engineering changes in the oil quality of seeds is inherently more difficult than modification of the protein composition because one needs to change the activity of an enzyme present in a complex pathway of metabolism, rather than producing a protein that has no metabolic function. The first attempts to change the oil composition of seeds are concentrating not on the change of enzyme activity, but on the change in content of the proteinaceous cofactor, acyl carrier protein (ACP).

REFERENCES

Altenbach, S.B., K.W. Pearson, F.W. Leung, and S.S.M. Sun. 1987. Cloning and sequence analysis of a cDNA encoding a Brazil nut protein exceptionally rich in methionine. *Plant Mol. Biol.* **8:** 239.

Sun, S.S.M., S.B. Altenbach, and F.W. Leung. 1987a. Properties, biosynthesis and processing of a sulfur-rich protein in Brazil nut (*Bertholletia excelsa* H.B.K.). *Eur. J. Biochem.* **162:** 477.

Sun, S.S.M., F.W. Leung, and J.C. Tomic. 1987b. Brazil nut (*Bertholletia excelsa* H.B.K.) proteins: Fractionation, composition, and identification of a sulfur-rich protein. *J. Agric. Food Chem.* **35:** 232.

Expression of Bacterial Chitinase in Plants

J.R. Bedbrook, J. Jones, T. Suslow, and P. Dunsmuir

Advanced Genetic Sciences, Inc., Oakland, California 94608

Chitinases, hydrolytic enzymes that degrade chitin, are found in a wide spectrum of organisms, including insects (Chen et al. 1982), nematodes, yeast and many other fungal and bacterial species (Elango et al. 1982), and higher plants. With the exception of bacteria and higher plants, the chitinase enzyme occurs together with its substrate chitin, an N-acetylglucosamine polymer, and is thought to be functional in growth, development, and differentiation. In higher plants, where there is no detectable chitin, chitinase is thought to serve a defense function. This notion is consistent with the observation that chitinase activity is induced by pathogen invasion and that many fungal plant pathogens and opportunistic saprophytes have chitin as a major cell-wall component. Chitinases have been shown to degrade fungal pathogen cell walls in vitro (Pegg and Young 1982), to be potent inhibitors of fungal growth (Schlumbaum et al. 1987), and to be nematicidal on some species of plant-parasitic nematodes (Miller and Sands 1977). The purpose of our experiments is to attempt to produce sufficiently high levels of bacterial chitinase in plants to investigate whether such plants have enhanced resistance to fungal diseases.

The Chitinase Genes of *Serratia marcescens*

We have isolated two nonhomologous genes, *chiA* and *chiB*, that encode distinct chitinase activities in *Serratia marcescens* QMB1466 (Jones et al. 1986). The *chiA* gene specifies a 58-kD protein, and the *chiB* gene specifies a 52-kD peptide. The nucleotide sequence of the *chiA* gene has been determined. Experiments in which the wild type and an isogenic *chiA* mutant strain of *S. marcescens* were compared for their ability to inhibit *Fusarium oxysporum* strongly indicate that the *chiA* gene is a major factor in the ability of *S. marcescens* to inhibit fungal growth, both in fungal spore elongation studies in vitro and in greenhouse tests of *F. oxysporum* infection on peas (Jones et al. 1986).

chiA Gene Expression in Plant Cells

The coding region from the *chiA* gene was fused to the promoter and 3' polyadenylation region of the *Agrobacterium tumefaciens* nopaline synthase gene, and the resulting construct was introduced into tobacco cells (Taylor et al. 1987). Site-directed mutagenesis of specific nucleotides surrounding the initiating AUG of the coding sequence in this chimeric gene resulting in the optimal −3 and +4 nucleotide composition (Kozak 1986) produced up to an eightfold increase in the amount of chitinase protein detected in transformed plant tissue. Analysis of the *chiA* mRNA indicated that these nucleotides also affected mRNA levels. At least 50% of the chitinase protein produced in transformed tobacco cells was the same molecular weight as the *S. marcescens* secreted protein.

High-level Expression of *chiA* Protein in Plants

The *S. marcescens chiA* gene was fused to a small subunit (*rbcS*) gene promoter and to two different chlorophyll *a/b* binding protein (*cab*) gene promoters from petunia. The resulting constructs were introduced into tobacco cells and used to generate multiple independent transgenic tobacco plants (J. Jones et al., in prep.). On average, the *rbcS/chiA* fusion gave rise to fourfold more *chiA* mRNA than either *cab/chiA* fusion. In those transformants showing the highest level of *chiA* expression, the *chiA* protein accumulated to about 0.2% of total soluble leaf protein. Even in plants showing the highest levels of chitinase expression, no detrimental effects on plant growth and development were associated with the high-expression phenotype.

Activity of *chiA* Protein in Plants

The possibility that the *chiA* protein is being processed in the plant secretory pathway makes it essential to determine whether the expression of this protein in plant tissue leads to increased chitinase enzyme activity. Protein was extracted from homozygous *chiA* individuals, as well as vector-transformed individuals as controls. Chitinase activity was assayed using the radioactive chitin procedure of Molano et al. (1977). The results of these experiments show that control transgenic plants do not have levels of chitinase activity significantly higher than untransformed plants. *chiA* transgenic plants have signficantly higher levels of chitinase than the controls do. The magnitude of the increase corresponds to an additional 30% over endogenous-induced activity. The observed activity parallels activity observed in reconstruction experiments in which purified *chiA* protein (prepared from *Escherichia coli* cells that carry the *chiA* gene) is added to the extracts from untransformed plant tissue.

DISCUSSION

A bacterial chitinase gene, *chiA*, can be expressed at high levels in plants. The protein produced retains the same apparent level of enzymatic activity when compared with that found in bacteria. The observed molecular weight of the protein in plant tissue indicates that it is correctly processed by plant cells. We are investigating the cellular location of the processed chitinase product. Our present work involves testing *chiA* transgenic plants, which are expressing significant levels of chitinase for their tolerance to various fungal plant pathogens. We are futher investigating the simultaneous expression of the *S. marcescens chiB*-gene product because the *chiA*- and *chiB*-gene products appear to have a synergistic effect on chitinase hydrolysis. The ultimate aim of our work is to develop crop plants with increased tolerance to chitin containing pathogens and pests.

REFERENCES

Chen, A., R. Mayer, and J. DeLoach. 1982. Purification and characterization of chitinase from the stable fly, *Stomoxys calcitrans*. *Arch. Biochem.* **216:** 314.

Elango, N., J. Correa, and E. Cabib. 1982. Secretory character of yeast chitinase. *J. Biol. Chem.* **257:** 1398.

Jones, J., K. Grady, T. Suslow, and J. Bedbrook. 1986. Isolation and characterization of genes encoding two distinct chitinase enzymes from *Serratia marcescens*. *EMBO J.* **5:** 467.

Kozak, M. 1986. Point mutations define a sequence flanking the AUG initiator codon that modulates translation by eucaryotic ribosomes. *Cell* **44:** 283.

Miller, P. and D. Sands. 1977. Effects of hydrolytic enzymes in plant-parasitic nematodes. *J. Nematol.* **9:** 192.

Molano, J., A. Duran, and E. Cabib. 1977. A rapid and sensitive assay for chitinase using tritiated chitin. *Ann. Biochem.* **83:** 648.

Pegg, G. and D. Young. 1982. Purification and characterization of chitinase enzymes from healthy and Verticillum infected tomato plants and from *V. albo-atrum*. *Physiol. Plant Pathol.* **21:** 389.

Schlumbaum, A., F. Mauch, U. Vogeli, and T. Boller. 1987. Plant chitinases are potent inhibitors of fungal growth. *Nature* **324:** 365.

Taylor, J., J. Jones, S. Sandler, G. Mueller, J. Bedbrook, and P. Dunsmuir. 1987. Optimizing the expression of a chimeric gene in plant cells. *Mol. Gen. Genet.* **210:** 572.

Maize Breeding and Seed Product Development

N.M. Frey, R.L. McConnell, and D.N. Duvick

Pioneer Hi-Bred International, Inc., Johnston, Iowa 50131

Regulations for the testing and use of genetically engineered plants must be developed on the basis of a knowledge of the existing seed business. The development and production of new seeds occur in the field, not in the laboratory and factory. Thus, regulatory procedures and perspectives need to appreciate the biological considerations that differentiate seed products from chemical or pharmaceutical products. Those regulations must also recognize differences in profitability of seed products relative to chemical or pharmaceutical products. My goal is to present a biological perspective of the seed business as it has been developed and as it exists today. I will also share some examples of profitability by seed product line to illustrate the differences in profitability that exist among seed products. I hope that perspective will be useful for our discussion of regulatory requirements for future genetically engineered seed products. Some may say that a regulatory framework exists, but the coordinated framework of June 1986 (Office of Science and Technology Policy 1986) fails to define the regulatory requirements that seed companies may face when farmers plant millions of acres of genetically engineered seeds to produce agricultural products for food, feed, and industrial markets that exist in the 1990s and beyond. To date, the regulatory debate has focused on small-scale field experiments of little relevance to seed product development requirements.

SUMMARY AND DISCUSSION

Until the 1980s, seed product development has been synonymous with plant breeding. The hybrid maize seed industry developed following George Shull's (1909) publication on the pure line method of corn breeding. Maize breeders have applied their skills in breeding, selection, and testing to improve maize performance fourfold since 1930. Maize breeding has, in fact, resulted in a genetic gain of approximately 1% per year in yield from 1930 through 1980 (Duvick 1979, 1983), and today, those same rates of gain appear to be accruing.

The maize breeder has relied on sexual crossing of elite breeding lines, followed by genetic recombination during several generations of self-pollination to develop new inbred lines that are suitable parents of commercial maize hybrids. The techniques that maize breeders use today are similar to those used by George Shull in 1909, but the scale and sophistication of the breeding effort are much greater. I will describe the maize breeding effort at a typical Pioneer maize breeding station to illustrate the process of maize seed product development today.

Pioneer currently has 25 maize breeding stations in the United States and Canada. A typical station will have 20,000 rows of nursery devoted to the development of new inbred lines, that is, the parents of hybrid seed products. In addition to this breeding nursery, the station will have a total of 12,000–20,000 yield test plots grown in ten or more locations to evaluate yield potential and agronomic adaptation of new hybrids compared to those hybrids currently being sold. Many of these yield test locations are in farmers' fields of corn, that is, we may have 1 to 10 acres of plots within a farmer's corn field of 40 or 100 or more acres.

Testing at multiple locations is crucial to seed product development. We are looking for maize hybrids that have stable performance across a number of growing environments. Maize breeders describe such hybrids as having low genotype by environment interaction.

To identify an elite commercial maize hybrid, yield testing will span 4 or more years, with each successive year of testing being more rigorous. If a hybrid reaches precommercial status, testing may expand to as many as 12 stations and five locations per station over a 2-year period. During the first year as a precommercial hybrid, foundation seed will be produced for the hybrid's parents, and a small quantity of hybrid seed (~250–400 units) will be produced in an isolated field. That hybrid seed will be distributed to the marketing regions for use in their on-farm strip-testing program. If performance of the new hybrid is good, up to 250,000 acres of the hybrid may be grown by farmers in the first year of introduction.

Pioneer alone sells over 80 hybrids in the United States. In 1987, 9 new hybrids were released, and another 13 precommercial hybrids were being strip tested and readied for release.

Forty other hybrids were in the first year of precommercial status, which includes initial hybrid production and foundation seed increase.

I have provided this detail on hybrid maize breeding, testing, and product sale to highlight the biological realities in seed product development. There is little parallel with chemical pesticide development. One herbicide may be suitable for use in corn production anywhere in the United States. No corn hybrid will be usable over such a broad geographic area. Some hybrids are broadly adapted and may be grown on millions of acres. Others are very narrowly adapted and may only be grown on perhaps 40,000 acres. Regulatory requirements (and costs) must recognize the requirements for seed product development, that is, wide-area testing to assess its competitiveness and stability of performance relative to existing seed products, and the opportunity to recover regulatory costs through seed sales. Seed products with low margins or with low volume sales will not support significant regulatory costs. For example, corn has a gross margin before tax of perhaps $6 per acre planted, while hybrid sorghum and soybean varieties return less than 50 cents per acre planted in gross margin. Regulatory costs will have to be consistent with profit potential if gene transfer technology is to be applied for improvement of a given crop.

The regulatory requirements should recognize that maize breeders have been exploiting genetic recombination in thousands of breeding populations for over 75 years, and no adverse environmental impact has occurred. Maize has not become a problem weed, nor has feed quality changed significantly.

Obviously, genetic engineering of plants will allow genetic recombinants not yet achieved by sexual crossing and selection. Some new gene introductions will pose new questions not only about efficacy as a seed product, but also about safety, because most agronomic produce will enter the food chain. The coordinated framework was developed to ensure that the application of recombinant DNA to crop improvement (as well as other applications) does not result in undesired consequences to the environment.

Discussions surrounding the questions of environmental release often project a sense that genetically engineered organisms are totally new and therefore the consequences of environmental release are totally unpredictable. It is important to remember that a genetically engineered corn plant will contain perhaps 20,000 uncharacterized genes plus 1 character-ized gene. Our experience in breeding, testing, and reproduc-ing maize plants before genetic engineering, that is, those with 20,000 uncharacterized genes, should be drawn upon extensive-ly as we look to regulate genetically engineered maize.

We must begin considering how to go from the small, isolat-ed, and very expensive field tests of genetically engineered plants, currently being conducted by a handful of companies, to millions of acres of crop production from genetically engineered seeds. Seed product development cannot occur within a few acres of fenced and closely monitored plots. Product develop-ment must occur in farmers' fields where important agronomic traits can be evaluated. What is the next step following an initial field test of a genetically engineered plant? Can we then turn the small amount of harvested seed over to plant breeders and begin the 3–10 years of product development required? That is what will be needed if American agriculture is to ex-ploit the opportunities that we all hope genetic engineering will bring.

REFERENCES

Duvick, D.N. 1979. Changes in productivity, maturity, and resistance to diseases and insects of U.S. corn hybrids grown during the past 45 years. In *Proceedings of the 10th Meeting of Eucarpia Corn and Sorghum Section.* Varna, Bulgaria.
———. 1983. Genetic contributions to yield gains of U.S. hybrid maize 1980–1980. *ASA Spec. Publ.* **7:** 15.
Office of Science and Technology Policy. 1986. Coordinated framework for regulation of biotechnology. Part II. *Federal Register* **51(123):** 23302.
Shull, G.H. 1909. A pure line method of corn breeding. *Proc. Am. Breeders' Assoc.* **5:** 51.

Evaluation of Genetically Engineered Plants

P.J. Dale and R.B. Flavell

Institute of Plant Science Research, Cambridge Laboratory
Cambridge CB2 2LQ, England

The modification of crops through the production of transgenic plants requires the identification of suitable characters for improvement. Many of the objectives of genetic engineering are already those of conventional breeding programs: resistance to disease, pests, and environmental stress; improved quality and quantity of harvestable yield; and reduced costs by more efficient use of inputs such as fertilizer. The improvement of crops by genetic engineering will more often give the genetic raw materials for a conventional breeding program than provide a marketable plant directly.

The rate of progress will depend on the identification and isolation of relevant genes, the ease of insertion of those genes into crop plants, and their stable expression and inheritance. There is progress in the isolation of genes conferring resistance to herbicides, viruses, and insects and their evaluation in transgenic plants. For example, at the Institute of Plant Science Research (IPSR; formerly, the Plant Breeding Institute [PBI]), we have recently created resistance to cucumber mosaic virus by expressing viral satellite RNA in transgenic tobacco (Harrison et al. 1987). We have also been concentrating on manipulating glutenin seed storage proteins with a view to inserting them into wheat to improve bread-making quality. To date, genes for glutenin proteins have been isolated and are expressed only in the endosperm of transgenic tobacco plants (Colot et al. 1988). The efficient introduction of genes into plants is determined primarily by two constraints: the ability of plant regeneration from cultured cells and the susceptibility of the crop to the transforming organism *Agrobacterium tumefaciens*. Dicotyledonous species are more amenable than monocotyledonous species in both respects. Introduced genes should be expressed at times and in tissues where their products are required. It might be detrimental to plant performance if genes are expressed to high levels in cells or tissues where they are not required. The choice of regulatory DNA is therefore important, and the genetic engineer requires a selection of promoters giving a variety of kinds of gene expression.

Data on gene expression can be obtained from plants grown in a controlled environment room and greenhouse but will have direct relevance to agronomic conditions only when transgenic plants are exposed to the complex and changing environment of the field. Field-testing of transgenic plants will also give experience in risk assessment, procedures of release from containment, and their practicality. By building up a bank of experience of the case histories of carefully managed experiments, we can begin to exploit some of the potential of genetic engineering in crop plants. We are currently doing this at IPSR via laboratory, greenhouse, and field evaluation of potatoes transformed by cocultivation of tuber disks with *A. tumefaciens*. This is a collaborative project involving M.W. Bevan, R. Jefferson, R.B. Flavell, and E. Atkinson (molecular biology), S. Sheerman, H. McPartland, P.J. Dale (transformation/tissue culture), A.J. Thomson, G. Jellis (potato breeder/pathologist), and R. Johnson (Chairman of PBI Genetic Manipulation Safety Committee).

Field Trial of Transgenic Potatoes

Transgenic potato plants are being tested under field conditions in 1987 and 1988. The DNA construct inserted by *A. tumefaciens* contains variants of the promoter from patatin, the principal protein of potato tubers, linked to the reporter gene β-glucuronidase. In addition to learning about alien gene regulation by this promoter during development, the trial should allow assessment of any attendant effects of the transformation process on plant morphology and yield, including those from somatic (somaclonal) variation and the presence of the neomycin phosphotransferase II gene, which enables kanamycin-resistant transformed cells to be selected.

The release from containment of genetically engineered organisms in the United Kingdom is dealt with by the Advisory Committee on Genetic Manipuation (ACGM). This is part of the Health and Safety Executive of the Department of Employment. The ACGM has issued guidelines for risk assessment and notification, and a response to these forms the basis of the request to release the plants into the environment. In line with ACGM requirements, the case for a field trial had to be considered first by an internal Institute Genetic Manipulation Safety

Committee for their assessment and approval. The stages in the submission are outlined in Table 1, along with an approximate time scale. Eight months elapsed from beginning preparation of the case to planting the trial. Many factors were considered in the submission, for example, location of the trial with respect to other potato plots; frequencies of outpollination; whether the trial should be fenced; the structure of the inserted DNA; the storage characteristics of harvested tubers; the method of disposal of leaves and tubers after sampling; the method of planting, weed control, and harvesting; and management of the trial after harvest.

Approximately 80 independently transformed plants were replicated along with untransformed controls to give almost 2000 plants in the field. The DNA inserted into potato was from potato and *Escherichia coli* and was nonhazardous, but various procedures for the handling and restriction of transgenic plant material are being evaluated in response to the ACGM recommendations.

The cultivations up to planting were done by machinery, but

Table 1 Procedure and Time Scale to Achieve the Go-ahead for the Field Trial of Transgenic Potatoes

Date	Details
1986	
October	Preparation of background papers.
November	First draft of case to PBI GM safety committee. Redrafts.
December	Approval by PBI GM safety committee. Submission to ACGM.
1987	
January	
February	PBI presentation of case to ACGM and discussions.
March	Broad approval received from ACGM subject to a satisfactory response from PBI to various proposals.
April	Submission of PBI response to ACGM proposals. "Informed the community" of the submission; discussions with local environmental health officers. Press release.
May	Go-ahead from ACGM.
June	MAFF licence issued. Field planting.

Abbreviations: PBI, Plant Breeding Institute; GM, genetic manipulation; ACGM, Advisory Committee on Genetic Manipulation; MAFF, Ministry of Agriculture, Fisheries, and Foods.

planting, weed control, harvesting, and all sampling were done by hand. Machinery did not pass through the plot to avoid transporting plant material away from the trial area. Pollen dissemination was prevented by regular inspection and removal of flower buds. In practice, this was possible to achieve before the petals became visible by inspecting the plants every 1 or 2 days. The harvesting of berries was recommended but proved unnecessary, because flower bud removal was effective in preventing seed and berry formation. The trial area will be kept fallow for 1 year after use and will be inspected, cultivated, and sprayed as necessary to remove ground-keeper tubers.

CONCLUSION

To take up opportunities from genetic engineering of crop plants, increasingly it will be necessary to test the expression and regulation of introduced genes under standard agronomic conditions. Refinement of the procedures of risk assessment will depend heavily on the experience of field assessment gained over the next few years. For the opportunities from genetic engineering to be taken up, it is vital that in the light of scientific evidence, experiments are given calm and careful consideration, case by case.

REFERENCES

Colot, V., L.S. Robert, T.A. Kavanagh, M.W. Bevan, and R.D. Thompson. 1988. Localisation of sequences in wheat endosperm protein genes which confer tissue-specific expression in tobacco. *EMBO J.* **16:** 3559.

Harrison, B.D., M.A. Mayo, and D.C. Baulcombe. 1987. Virus resistance in transgenic plants that express cucumber mosaic virus satellite RNA. *Nature* **328:** 799.

Engineering Insect and Herbicide-resistant Crops

J. Leemans

Plant Genetic Systems N.V., B-9000 Gent, Belgium

Gene-transfer techniques have been used to introduce two traits of agronomic importance into several plant species. Evaluations of these new plant varieties have indicated that chimeric genes for insect and herbicide resisitance are expressed and produce adequate levels of protection under field conditions.

RESULTS AND DISCUSSION
Engineering Lepidoptera Resistance in Plants

Commerical preparations of spores of the bacterium *Bacillus thuringiensis* (*Bt*) occupy a prominent place in the field of insect biocontrol. They combine high insect toxicity with environmental safety. *Bt* does not affect nontarget insects and is completely nontoxic to vertebrates. The crystalline inclusions that are produced upon sporulation contain insecticidal proteins that affect the midgut epithelium of sensitive insects.

We have used *Agrobacterium*-mediated transfer DNA to express several modified genes derived from the Lepidoptera-specific *bt2* gene in tobacco and potato. The expression of genes that contained the amino-terminal half of *bt2* fused to the *neo* gene was particularly successful. These encode fusion proteins that exhibit both insect toxicity and neomycin phosphotransferase activity. The latter was used to select cells that expressed substantial amounts of insecticidal protein (Vaeck et al. 1987).

High toxicity, resulting in 80–100% mortality of *Manduca sexta* larvae, was observed in tobacco plants expressing fusion proteins or a truncated *bt2* gene (Table 1). None of the plants transformed with the full-length *bt2* gene produced insect-killing activity. Also, potato plants transformed with a fusion gene or a truncated *bt2* gene exhibited significant insecticidal activity. Greenhouse experiments revealed that the transgenic plants are protected against insect-feeding damage. They showed by limited damage, restricted to feeding areas of a few

Table 1 Insect-killing Activity on *M. sexta* in a 6-day Feeding Assay

Bt gene[a]	Ti plasmid	Percentage of plants causing a mortality						Total no. of plants
		0–20%	20–40%	40–60%	60–80%	80–95%	100%	
Tobacco								
Bt:NPT fusion	pGS1151	46	17	11	11	11	3	35
Bt:NPT fusion	pGS1152	8	16	4	16	20	36	25
Bt2	pGS1161	92	8	0	0	0	0	13
Bt truncated	pGS1163	13	27	0	3	33	27	15
Potato								
Bt:NPT fusion	pGS1152	0	19	13	25	25	19	16
Bt truncated	pGS1163	35	19	16	13	3	13	16

Recombinant Ti plasmids are described in Vaeck et al. (1987).
[a]NPT, neomycin phosphotransferase.

square millimeters, whereas control plants were entirely consumed within 10 days. *Bt* protein levels in the insect-resistant plants ranged from 7 to 40 ng/mg total protein.

Prospects for Engineering Broad Insect Resistance
Most Lepidoptera- and Diptera-specific *Bt* toxins are 130–140 kD and are, in fact, "protoxins" which, after solubilization in the insect midgut, are proteolytically processed toward smaller actively toxic polypeptides of ±60 kD. Interestingly, the Coleoptera toxin from *B. thuringiensis* var. *tenebrionis* (Bt13) appears as a naturally processed toxin in the crystal (Höfte et al. 1987). Despite their clearly distinct spectrum of insecticidal activity, these three classes of *Bt* proteins are members of the same family of structurally related proteins and may use a similar mechanism to interact with the insect cells. The detailed knowledge about the structural properties of different *Bt* proteins may lead to an understanding of the parameters that determine their specificity. Ultimately, this information may be used to construct new types of insecticidal proteins with improved activity or a broader host range.

Herbicide Resistance
We have engineered resistance against the nonselective herbicides phosphinothricin (a potent inhibitor of glutamine synthetase [Bayer et al. 1972]) and bialaphos. Bialaphos is produced by *Streptomyces hygroscopicus* and consists of phosphinothricin and two L-alanine residues (Ogawa et al. 1973). Phosphinothricin is chemically synthesized (BASTA[R], Hoechst AG), whereas bialaphos is produced by fermentation of *S. hygroscopicus* (Herbiace[R], Meiji Seika Ltd.).

Recently, we have isolated a bialaphos resistance gene (*bar*) from *S. hygroscopicus*. This gene encodes a phosphinothricin acetyltransferase (Thompson et al. 1987) that acetylates the free amino-terminal group of phosphinothricin and thereby prevents autotoxicity of phosphinothricin in *Streptomyces*. We have expressed the *bar* gene driven by the cauliflower mosaic virus (CaMV) 35S promoter in transgenic tomato, potato, and tobacco. These plants showed high levels of resistance against field-dose applications of the commercial formulations of phosphinothricin and bialaphos under greenhouse conditions. The glutamine synthetase of transgenic plants was not affected by the herbicide treatment (DeBlock et al. 1987). F_1 progeny of two transgenic tobacco lines that expressed the resistance gene

Table 2 Effect of Herbicide Sprays on BASTA[R] resistant Tobacco

Tobacco line	Phosphinothricin dose (kg/ha)			
	0	1	2	4
Control SR1	20.45	0[a]	0[a]	0[a]
N78–107	23.80	24.20	24.20	24.30
N78–108	20.00	23.10	24.05	23.65

Measurement of the length of the largest leaf (cm).
[a]All plants destroyed by the herbicide.

were tested in the field. Phosphinothricin was applied 20 days after transfer to the field at 1, 2, and 4 kg/hectare (ha) as a commercial formulation of BASTA[R].

Table 2 shows that both transgenic tobacco lines were fully resistant against a postemergent application of BASTA[R]. These plants did not show any symptoms of herbicidal activity even when phosphinothricin was applied at a dose of 4 kg/ha. Normal field applications are 0.5–1.5 kg/ha. Phosphinothricin acetyltransferase was expressed at a level of 0.001% of total extracted protein in N78-108 and at 0.1% in N78-107 (DeBlock et al. 1987). We conclude that the resistance gene is expressed in N78-107 at at least 100-fold above the level required for exhibiting complete resistance.

In conclusion, phosphinothricin resistance has been confirmed under field conditions in transgenic tobacco. The successful engineering of this detoxifying enzyme will be largely independent from the plant species used. We expect it to be useful to engineer resistance into major crops such as sugarbeet and oil seed rape.

REFERENCES

Bayer, E., K.H. Gugel, K. Hagele, H. Hagenmaier, S. Jessipow, W.A. Koning, and H. Zahner. 1972. Stoffwechselprodukte von Mikroorganismen. Phosphinothricin und phosphinothricyl-alanyl-alanin. *Helv. Chim. Acta* **55**: 224.

DeBlock, M., J. Botterman, M. Vandewiele, J. Dockx, C. Thoen, V. Gosselé, N.R. Movva, C. Thompson, M. Van Montagu, and J. Leemans. 1987. Engineering herbicide resistance in plants by expression of a detoxifying enzyme. *EMBO J.* **6**: 2513.

Höfte, H., J. Seurinck, A. Van Houtven, and M. Vaeck. 1987. Nucleotide sequence of a gene encoding an insecticidal protein of *Bacillus thuringiensis* var. *tenebrionis* toxic against Coleoptera. *Nucleic Acids Res.* **15**: 7183.

Ogawa, Y., T. Tsuruoka, S. Inouye, and T. Niida. 1973. Studies on a new antibiotic SF-1293. *Sci. Rep. Meiji Seika Kaisha* **13**: 42.

Thompson, C., N.R. Movva, R. Tizard, R. Crameri, J.E. Davies, M. Lauwereys, and J. Botterman. 1987. Characterization of the herbicide-resistance gene *bar* from *Streptomyces hygroscopicus*. *EMBO J.* **6:** 2519.

Vaeck, M., A. Reynaerts, H. Höfte, S. Jansens, M. De Beuckeleer, C. Dean, M. Zabeau, M. Van Montagu, and J. Leemans. 1987. Transgenic plants protected from insect attack. *Nature* **328:** 33.

Field Testing Genetically Engineered Plants

TOMATOES

R.T. Fraley

Monsanto Company (BB3B), St. Louis, Missouri 63198

The field testing of genetically engineered plants represents an important step in the commercialization of plant biotechnology research. In view of recent research breakthroughs, increased public awareness, and the existence of new regulatory policies, such tests have undoubtedly taken on greater significance than deserved. It is important to remember that many of the first tests that have been conducted were not with commercial cultivars and that several years of plant breeding efforts, field evaluations, and scale-up lie ahead before improved crops will be marketed. At the same time, however, the technology is developing faster than most realize, and already issues such as regulatory costs and registration timelines are becoming key concerns to companies attempting to develop improved genetically engineered crops.

In 1987, the Monsanto Company carried out field evaluations on three different classes of genetically engineered tomato plants that carried newly introduced genes for conferring tolerance to tobacco mosaic virus (TMV), lepidopteran insects, and Roundup[R] herbicide, respectively. The results of these experiments are discussed below.

Field Test Background

Transgenic tomatoes (VF36) for the field test were produced using a Ti plasmid-based transformation system as described previously (Fraley et al. 1986). TMV-tolerant plants contained a chimeric construct encoding the TMV coat protein gene under control of the cauliflower mosaic virus (CaMV) 35S promoter (Abel et al. 1986). Insect-tolerant plants contained the *Bacillus thuringiensis* (*Bt*) insect control protein as described recently (Fischhoff et al. 1987). Roundup-tolerant tomato plants were produced that carried a petunia cDNA clone encoding an altered 5-enolpyruvylshikimate-3-phosphate synthase (EPSPS; Shah et al. 1986). Southern hybridization analysis of over 70 trangenic tomatoes and their progeny confirmed the absence of *Agrobacterium tumefaciens* contamination; genetic analysis confirmed the stable inheritance of all three inserted traits.

The site chosen for the field test was a farm located 3 miles outside the farming community of Jerseyville, Illinois. The test plot was well-drained and was not located near a flood plain or tomato production areas. The site was fenced to protect the plants from damage by animals. The local community and state officials were briefed in advance; as expected, there was strong local support for the tests. Over 9000 tomato transplants were planted between the first and third weeks of June; agronomic conditions were chosen that closely paralleled commercial practices. The site was monitored throughout the season to determine possible effects of the transgenic plants on normal insect populations—none were observed. The plants were allowed to flower and all fruit was collected prior to color break to minimize attractiveness to birds and rodents. After sampling, excess fruit was oven dried on site and later incinerated. Upon termination of the experiment, the tomato plants were plowed under. The site will be monitored next spring and any volunteer tomatoes will be controlled by herbicide application or mechanical cultivation.

Field Test Results

Insect-tolerant Plants. The insect-tolerant plants containing the *Bt* gene were infested with egg masses of *Manduca sexta* (tobacco hornworm) and *Heliothis zea* (tomato fruitworm). The level of insect control observed in the field tests was generally superior to that observed in growth chamber experiments. Under conditions where control plants were totally defoliated by the hornworm infestation, tomato plants containing the *Bt* gene suffered no agronomic damage. Similar results were obtained with control and *Bt*-containing tomato plants following natural or inoculated infestations by tomato fruitworm. Fruit damage on control plots was 17–23%, whereas fruit damage on *Bt* plants was only 4–9%. The excellent insect control observed under field conditions may be a result of using egg mass inoculations instead of young larvae as in the growth chamber experiments; this may have allowed more effective control at early stages in insect development. It is also possible that the feeding-deterrent effects associated with the *Bt* insecticidal protein are more pronounced under natural field conditions.

Virus-tolerant Plants. The TMV-tolerant plants were hand inoculated with 10–40 µg/ml of TMV (U1 strain) at different intervals after transplanting. In all cases, 100% of the control plants exhibited virus symptoms and tested positive for the presence of TMV. In contrast, less than 5% of the transgenic tomatoes containing the chimeric coat protein gene displayed symptoms. Where symptoms did appear on the transgenic plants, they were quite mild and were restricted to the inoculated leaves. Biochemical tests confirmed the lack of systemic spread of the virus in the transgenic plants. In the absence of virus pressure, the transgenic tomato plants expressing TMV coat protein yielded comparably to controls, indicating that the presence of the coat protein does not affect plant growth. Interestingly, the transgenic plants showed no yield reduction after virus infection, whereas the control plants suffered 23–33% yield losses. This result was somewhat surprising, since the U1 TMV strain caused only mild symptoms on the control plants. These results may indicate, as many plant pathologists suspect, that "subclinical" levels of viral diseases in plants may cause significant but generally unobserved yield reductions.

Roundup-herbicide-tolerant Plants. The Roundup-tolerant tomatoes containing an overexpressed mutant petunia *EPSPS* gene also yielded comparably to controls in the absence of herbicide treatment, indicating that alteration of *EPSPS* levels has no effect on plant growth. Twenty-two independently derived transgenic tomato lines were evaluated in the test; the best plants survived Roundup applications of over 1 lb/acre; in contrast, control plants were completely killed at this rate. The treated transgenic plants displayed excellent vegetative tolerance, but showed reduced and delayed flowering relative to unsprayed controls. Given the extreme sensitivity of tomatoes to damage by Roundup exposure, the dramatic increase in tolerance observed in the field results is extremely encouraging and indicates that tolerance to commercial rates (0.5–1 lb/acre) should be achievable.

SUMMARY
Although the commercial significance of this year's field tests will only be determined after much additional evaluation, several important observations are noted here: (1) Field experiments were carried out with local community support; (2) there were no adverse effects of engineered plants on the test-site environment; (3) introduced traits did not affect plant growth or reduce yield; and (4) field performance was as good as or better than greenhouse tests.

It will be important that the process for evaluating field testing of genetically engineered plants recognizes and responds quickly to the need for testing of additional plants at multiple locations. It will also be important in subsequent evaluations that normal agronomic practices be employed in field tests, including completion of crop reproduction cycles and testing in normal production areas. Finally, it is critical that regulatory requirements dealing with the commercialization of genetically engineered plants be formulated in a fashion that recognizes the inherent low risk of the technology and that does not draw undue attention to the particular biotechnology process used to improve plants.

REFERENCES

Abel, P.P., R.S. Nelson, B. De, N. Hoffmann, S.G. Rogers, R.T. Fraley, and R.N. Beachy. 1986. Delay of disease development in transgenic plants that express the tobacco mosaic virus coat protein gene. *Science* **232**: 738.

Fischhoff, D.A., K.S. Bowdish, F.J. Perlak, P.G. Marrone, S.M. McCormick, J.G. Niedermeyer, D.A. Dean, K. Kusano-Kretzmer, E.J. Mayer, D.E. Rochester, S.G. Rogers, and R.T. Fraley. 1987. Insect tolerant transgenic tomato plants. *Bio/Technology* **5**: 807.

Fraley, R.T., S.G. Rogers, and R.B. Horsch. 1986. Genetic transformation in higher plants. *Crit. Rev. Plant Sci.* **4**: 1.

Shah, D.M., R.B. Horsch, H.J. Klee, G.M. Kishore, J.A. Winter, N.E. Tumer, C.M. Hironaka, P.R. Sanders, C.S. Gasser, S. Aykent, N.R. Siegel, S.G. Rogers, and R.T. Fraley. 1986. Engineering herbicide tolerance in transgenic plants. *Science* **233**: 478.

EPA Regulation of Genetically Engineered Plants

P.A. Roberts

Office of General Counsel, U.S. Environmental Protection Agency
Washington, D.C. 20460

The U.S. Environmental Protection Agency (EPA) is one of
several federal agencies involved in regulating products of
biotechnology. As used in the June 26, 1986, "Coordinated
Framework for Regulation of Biotechnology" (51 Fed. Reg.
23302), the term biotechnology is broadly defined as "the application of biological systems and organisms to technical and
industrial processes."[1] Such a definition clearly encompasses
genetically engineered plants. Whether these altered plants
will be regulated by the EPA is therefore a question of how,
where, and for what purpose the plants will be used.

At this time, most of the EPA's regulatory effort involving
products of biotechnology is pursuant to its authority under the
Federal Insecticide, Fungicide, and Rodenticide Act (FIFRA), 7
U.S.C. 136 et seq, and the Toxic Substances Control Act
(TSCA), 15 U.S.C. 2601 et seq. FIFRA authorizes the EPA to
regulate the distribution, sale, and use of pesticides; TSCA authorizes the EPA to review "chemical substances" and "mix-
tures" of chemical substances not regulated under other
statutes in order to identify and, if necessary, regulate potential hazards and exposures related to these substances.

Most of this discussion will focus on regulation under
FIFRA because, as stated in the June 26 Coordinated Framework, the EPA's current thinking is that for the foreseeable future, most genetically engineered plants will be used for food,
food-related, or pesticidal purposes. These things are all exempt from TSCA by definition. Accordingly, at this time, the
EPA has no intent to regulate genetically engineered plants

---

[1]The definition of biotechnology was originally set out in the "Proposal for a
Coordinated Framework for Regulation of Biotechnology" (49 Fed. Reg. 50856
at 50906, December 31, 1984).

under TSCA.[2] However, "at this time" must be emphasized. Should a genetically engineered plant be developed for non-food/nonpesticidal purposes, the EPA would reassess its TSCA position in light of the expertise and regulatory mandates of other federal agencies.

As to pesticides, we have all read the headlines—"Potato Plant Produces Repellant;" "Corn Kills Worm." From a regulatory standpoint, these headlines raise two important questions: Is it a pesticide? If so, how will it be regulated?

The answer to the first question is fairly straightforward. Simply stated, if it acts like a pesticide or if it is intended to be used as a pesticide, under Section 2 of FIFRA, by definition, it is a pesticide. Here, the emphasis is on "by definition," and that leads to the second question.

The fact than an agent falls within the statutory definition of pesticide does not necessarily mean that it will be subjected to regulation under FIFRA. Section 25 allows the EPA to exempt from the requirements of FIFRA any pesticide determined to be adequately regulated by another federal agency or to be of a nature as to not require regulation.

In 1981, the EPA issued a regulation under Section 25, set out in the Code of Federal Regulations (CFR) at 40 CRF 162.5, that exempted all biological control agents, except certain microorganisms, from further regulation under FIFRA. Biological control agents include plants that have a pesticidal function. The EPA concluded at that time that these macroorganisms were adequately regulated by other federal agencies, such as the U.S. Department of Agriculture (USDA) and the U.S. Department of Interior. The EPA went on to say, however, that if the situation changed, it would have to reconsider its decision. This 1981 position was restated in the June 26 Coordinated Framework.

Recent technology has allowed the development of plants that have been engineered to incorporate or produce pesticidal agents that the plants do not contain naturally. Some of these pesticidal agents (e.g., *Bacillus thuringiensis* toxin) are the

[2]The June 26 Coordinated Framework lists two exceptions to this general rule (51 Fed. Reg. 23302 at 23324). First, if plant gene segments are intentionally incorporated into microorganisms, the microorganisms that contain those plant genes may be subject to TSCA, depending on how they are used. Second, a chemical extracted from a plant may be subject to TSCA, again depending on how it is used.

same as or similar to pesticides already regulated under FIFRA. Where, then, does the EPA stand on these new types of plants? Over the past year or two, the EPA has received a number of inquiries asking that very question. The following briefly summarizes the EPA's current thinking on this issue.

FIFRA is a comprehensive statute that provides the EPA with very broad authority to review the environmental impacts of pesticidal agents and, if necessary, to regulate them in order to protect man and the environment. It is therefore reasonable to conclude that the authors of FIFRA intended its authority to extend to all pesticidal agents, regardless of how they are packaged or transported into the environment. The real question then becomes, Could plants engineered to incorporate a pesticidal agent raise environmental and human health issues related to the pesticide component that warrant review under FIFRA, in addition to any review of the plant itself under other statutes? Without providing any specific answers, some of the issues that the EPA needs to consider include the following:

1. Given that many of these plants will be food crops for human consumption, what kinds of tolerances, if any, are required for residues of the pesticide component? (Under the Reorganization Plan of 1970 that established it, the EPA has the authority to set tolerances for pesticide residues in food and food crops.)
2. What is the likelihood and impact of transfer of genetic material from the pesticide component to other environmental niches, e.g., as in pollen-mediated transfer to other crops?
3. Does inclusion in a plant carrier impart different persistence or availability characteristics to the pesticide component that enhance its exposure potential for nontarget, and possibly endangered, species?

Certainly, most of these issues become more pressing when large-scale environmental applications are involved. In small-scale applications, the situation can usually be limited so as to eliminate or minimize these concerns. To date, the EPA has only considered small-scale situations.

The EPA has recently worked closely with the USDA on reviews of several small-scale uses of plants engineered to contain pesticidal agents. The two agencies have also informally agreed upon interim procedures for future joint reviews of small-scale field trials of such plants. This cooperative effort is working well and provides for thorough, simultaneous reviews that benefit from the expertise of both agencies and that satisfy the statutory mandates of both agencies. The EPA sees no immediate need to change this system.

However, once a producer decides on large-scale or commercial use of a plant that has been genetically engineered to produce its own pesticide—applications that have potential for substantial human or environmental exposure—it is difficult to see how the statute could be read so as to exclude the pesticide component from more formal review under FIFRA.

Genetically Modified Agricultural Crops: An FDA Perspective

J.H. Maryanski

Center for Food Safety and Applied Nutrition, Food and Drug
Administration, Washington, D.C. 20204

This year, tomato plants that were genetically modified by
recombinant DNA techniques for herbicide and pest resistance
were field tested for the first time. Programs to improve nutritional characteristics and other desirable traits of agricultural
crops are also in progress. Thus, it is timely to consider factors
that may affect the regulatory status of new food products and
the safety of the products for human health and the environment. This paper focuses on the role of the Food and Drug Administration (FDA) in protecting the public health, the laws
and regulations that apply to food, and some considerations
that pertain to the safety assessment of new food products.

The authority of the FDA, under the Federal Food, Drug,
and Cosmetic Act (the Act), over food and food ingredients cen-
ters on the product that is introduced into interstate commerce,
rather than on the method of manufacture. It is the primary
responsibility of the FDA to ensure a safe and wholesome food
supply for the nation. Under the leadership of Commissioner
Frank E. Young, the FDA is committed to a science-based
regulatory framework that will fully protect public health and
stimulate innovation. The general policies of the FDA concerning the application of new technology to food products (i.e., new
biotechnology) were published in the *Federal Register* (Office of
Science and Technology Policy 1986). The FDA proposed no
new procedures or requirements for regulated industry. The
laws and regulations under which the FDA approves products
place the burden of proof of safety on the manufacturer. Although there are no statutory provisions or regulations that address new technologies specifically, the FDA possesses extensive experience in the safety evaluation of products made by
traditional methods, and food products derived by new technologies can be adequately regulated within the framework of
the existing law. The administrative review of new products

will be based on the intended use of each product on a case-by-case basis.

Legal Statutes and Regulations

A discussion of genetically modified agricultural crops and the role of the FDA in assessing their safety must involve a consideration of the pertinent laws and regulations. Most issues concerning the safety of a food involve the application of the food adulteration provisions (Section 402), the food additive provisions (Section 409), or the color additive provisions (Section 706) of the Act. The food adulteration provisions provide, in part, that a food is adulterated if it bears or contains any poisonous or deleterious "added substance" that may render it injurious to health. Courts have agreed with the FDA's interpretation of this section that any substance that is not an inherent constituent of food may be regulated as an "added substance." Furthermore, if the quantity of a food constituent exceeds the amount that would normally be present because of some technological adjustment to the product, the excess quantity may also be viewed as an added substance.

The other statutory provisions of the Act used by the FDA in determining the safety of food and food ingredients are the food additive provisions (Sections 201[s] and 409) and the color additive provisions (Sections 201[t] and 706). The Act requires that substances employed to color food be used as prescribed by regulation and therefore requires premarket approval for color additives. The definition of a food additive (Section 201[s] of the Act) includes both artificial and natural substances and provides, in part, that the term food additive means any substance that, through its intended use, may become a component or affect the characteristics of any food, unless the substance is generally recognized as safe (GRAS) by qualified experts. Premarket approval is required for food additives, and industry frequently requests the FDA's opinion concerning GRAS status of a food product.

The procedural regulations of the FDA for GRAS food ingredients are described in the Code of Federal Regulations (21 CFR 170.30) and state that the FDA will review the GRAS status of ingredients of natural biological origin that have been widely used for nutrient properties and that have been signficantly altered by breeding and selection or by the manufacturing process. The FDA intends to review new methods of manufacture for food products by the same criteria used for products derived by traditional means. It is important to evaluate whether new methods result in changes in the chemical identity of the product, in the introduction into the food supply of new or altered levels of impurities, or in an increase in dietary exposure of consumers to the product that is not justified by available safety data. If the FDA finds that a food product manufactured by a new method has been altered significantly, the FDA will conclude either that the new product is also GRAS or that it is not GRAS and requires premarket approval under the food additive provisions of Section 409 of the Act.

Most traditional staple food is considered to be GRAS on the basis of a history of safe use prior to 1958. The central question to be considered when a food (e.g., tomato, carrot, wheat, beef, or eggs) is modified by chemical, physical, or biological processes is "Is the modified food or food ingredient still GRAS?" The question must focus on the commercial product and not on the process by which the product was derived.

Safety Assessment
The safety assessment of new food products should be stepwise, focusing on the chemical composition of the product (including impurities), the genetic modification employed, the nature of any microorganisms used to produce or modify the product, and its intended use in food. This information may then be used to establish appropriate toxicological requirements. This approach means that decisions concerning the use of new food products will be based on sound scientific principles.

The ability to transfer genetic information, including regulatory sequences that control gene expression, among diverse organisms may raise the potential for significant alterations to occur in the final food product. Because of this, the FDA encourages companies and individuals to consult with it in the early phase of research and development so that it may evaluate the significance of any change in the new food product.

DISCUSSION
In food and agriculture, much promise of new technologies is still to be realized. However, scientific developments are technically feasible or will be in the foreseeable future to enhance the essential amino acid content of food, such as corn, to minimize the production of unwanted metabolites at the level of

gene expression by antisense RNA and to introduce genes for herbicide resistance and other desirable properties into agricultural crops.

Nearly 15 years of research and commercial experience in recombinant DNA technology have demonstrated the safety and power of the methods of this new capability to modify genetic structure. This is clearly supported by a recent report (National Academy of Sciences 1987) that concluded, in part,

"There is no evidence that unique hazards exist either in the use of recombinant-DNA techniques or in the movement of genes between unrelated organisms."

"The risks associated with the introduction of recombinant DNA-engineered organisms are the same in kind as those associated with the introduction of unmodified organisms and organisms modified by other methods."

"Assessment of the risks of introducing recombinant DNA-engineered organisms into the environment should be based on the nature of the organism and the environment into which it is introduced, not on the method by which it was produced."

In this spirit, the FDA believes that new laws or regulations are not necessary to assess the safety of food products produced through new applications of biotechnology. The FDA intends to review products of new biotechnology on an individual basis by the same criteria used for products developed by traditional means, with particular emphasis on the nature of the genetically modified product and its intended use.

ACKNOWLEDGMENTS
The author thanks colleagues of the Food and Drug Administration, especially Mary Ann Danello, Henry I. Miller, and Gerad L. McCowin for their critical review of the manuscript.

REFERENCES
National Academy of Sciences. 1987. *Introduction of recombinant DNA-engineered organisms into the environment: Key issues.* National Academy Press, Washington, D.C.
Office of Science and Technology Policy. 1986. Coordinated framework for regulation of biotechnology. *Federal Register* **51**: 23302.

The NAS Policy Process: Examples in Biological Control and Organism Introductions

C.J. Gabriel[1] and P.B. Moses[2]

[1]Board on Basic Biology and [2]Board on Agriculture, National Research Council, Washington, D.C. 20418

The National Academy of Sciences (NAS) is a private, nonprofit honorary society of scientists who have distinguished themselves in research. The NAS was chartered by the U.S. Congress in 1863. Its dedication to the promotion of science and technology includes the responsibility to advise the federal government on scientific and technical issues. This mandate is carried out by the NAS operating branch, the National Research Council (NRC). NRC staff work together with advisory committees composed of NAS members and other leading scientists in studying policy components of all fields of science, engineering, and medicine.

Topics are divided among several NRC commissions and boards that cover diverse scientific disciplines. Each of these units has a standing committee of eminent scientists who guide its activities. In-house staff conduct the day-to-day operation of the units and their various science policy projects.

Activities dealing with agricultural biotechnology are handled by several boards, depending upon the policy focus. The Board on Agriculture has conducted a number of relevant studies over the past 5 years, including a recent comprehensive overview of problems in funding research, training researchers, and transferring new technologies and a report reviewing the peer review system within the U.S. Department of Agriculture's Agricultural Research Service (National Research Council 1987a,b). The Board on Basic Biology has published two reports this year that address special topics in agricultural biotechnology (National Academy of Sciences 1987a,b).

The Report of the Research Briefing Panel on Biological Control in Managed Ecosystems (National Academy of Sciences 1987a) was presented in a special briefing session to the U.S. President's science advisor and the director of the National Science Foundation. The panel's report has been influential to

Table 1 Selected Examples of Biological Controls

Component	Strategy		
	regulation of the pest population	exclusionary systems of protection	self-defense
Pest agent used against itself	**A** Pheromone gossypol to control pink bollworm in cotton	**B** Ice-minus strains of *Pseudomonas syringae* to exclude ice-nucleation-active strains from leaves of frost-sensitive plants	**C** Resistance to tobacco mosaic virus (TMV) in tobacco plants genetically engineered to express the coat-protein gene of TMV
Natural enemies and antagonists (classic biological control agents)	**D** *Bacillus thuringiensis* for control of certain caterpillars	**E** Toxin gene from *B. thuringiensis* expressed in *Pseudomonas* on corn roots for protection against certain soil insects	**F** Toxin gene from *B. thuringiensis* expressed in tobacco leaves for control of certain leaf-feeding caterpillars
Host plant or animal	**G** *Crotalaria* grown as a trap plant; root-knot nematode infects this plant but does not reproduce	**H** Dense sowings of cereal-grain crops to preempt establishment of weeds	**I** Genetic resistance to southern corn leaf blight in corn

The Research Briefing Panel (National Academy of Sciences 1987a) organized the broad subject of biocontrol into a grid. This new view recognizes three components and three strategies, giving nine types of biocontrol. A–I illustrate these with selected examples. Traditional biocontrol is confined largely to D (although many other examples could be given). However, all three strategies can be illustrated by the biocontrol agent *Bacillus thuringiensis*. Traditionally, preparations of *Bt* have been used against caterpillars and, more recently, blackflies and mosquitos. The active ingredient is a bacterial toxin which, when ingested by an insect, kills by lysing the gut cells (D). With recombinant DNA technology, the *Bt* toxin gene was transferred into and expressed in a common soil bacterium that colonizes corn roots (*Pseudomonas fluorescens*) (E) and in tobacco plants (F). When the toxin gene is expressed in its native *B. thuringiensis*, it regulates the pest population (strategy 1). When *B. thuringiensis* itself or the genetically engineered *P. fluorescens* are applied as microbial pesticides on plants, they mitigate insect attack by operating as an exclusionary system of protection (strategy 2). When the toxin gene is expressed in tobacco leaves, it provides the plant with a self-defense system (strategy 3). Recombinant DNA technology will undoubtedly yield other new uses of traditional biocontrol agents, as well as new agents (current examples in B and C).

97

the U.S. Department of Agriculture; in addition, copies have been distributed to the general public. This report, like other NAS research briefings on selected topics, surveyed the field's status and identified important research opportunities as well as current barriers to progress.

Biocontrol is a means of controlling a pest, using an organism detrimental to the pest. Traditionally, biocontrol has been viewed as a narrow area of agricultural research with limited applications. In light of new methodologies—molecular biology, computer modeling—biocontrol research should be refocused from the narrow traditional view to a broader view described by the briefing panel (Table 1). The new focus should expand the funding base directly available to biocontrol research, as well as increase the power and scope of biocontrol strategies.

The panel recommended several ways to advance the science and practice of biocontrol, calling for more basic research, with some redirection of existing resources, in part, to attract a greater number of well-qualified researchers. Important research areas include ecology of managed soils, organismal interactions, and molecular signals. The panel urged broader thinking in the research community—biocontrol is not a narrow field of applied biology. In that vein, the panel recommended interdisciplinary teams to solve complex problems. These had also been recommended by previous research briefing panels on agricultural biotechnology convened by the Board on Agriculture. The panel identified a critical need to efficiently move research out of the laboratory and into the field. Scientists tend to avoid this, considering it "not their job" or too high risk. On the other hand, one scientist cannot do it all, and often a product emphasis from industry is important.

New biocontrol agents created via recombinant DNA technology must be released into the environment to be of use. Regulatory concerns for both research and field testing have been problematic. The panel concluded that regulatory controls should be based on a product's properties, not on the process by which it was derived.

This point is the crux of the second study conducted by the Board on Basic Biology (National Academy of Sciences 1987b). A special committee convened by the NAS reviewed the relevant issues and produced a concise report explaining them at the layman's level. The conclusions of the panel encompass four points: (1) Unique hazards do not appear to be associated with either the use of recombinant DNA techniques or the transfer of genes between unrelated organisms. (2) The introduction into the environment of recombinant-DNA-engineered organisms poses risks no different from those associated with the introduction of unmodified organisms or organisms modified by other genetic techniques. (3) Assessment of risks should be based on the properties of the organism and the environment into which it will be introduced, not on the method by which the organism was modified. (4) The committee called upon the scientific community to provide guidance to both researchers and regulators for evaluating planned introductions of modified organisms from the ecological perspective.

The NAS considers the issue of introductions of genetically engineered organisms to be a pressing science policy concern and is proposing further studies that will clarify scientific aspects. In particular, science can address what properties of the organism and the environment should be considered when contemplating planned introductions and how regulations should be structured to reflect these properties.

ACKNOWLEDGMENTS
The authors acknowledge the invaluable contributions of their committee members and chairmen of each of the four National Academy of Sciences and National Research Council studies cited. In addition, the authors gratefully acknowledge the support of the Board on Basic Biology and the Board on Agriculture.

REFERENCES
National Academy of Sciences. 1987a. Report of the research briefing panel on biological control in managed ecosystems. Committee on Science, Engineering, and Public Policy. National Academy Press, Washington, D.C.
————. 1987b. *Introduction of recombinant DNA-engineered organisms into the environment: Key issues.* National Academy Press, Washington, D.C.
National Research Council. 1987a. *Agricultural biotechnology: Strategies for national competitiveness.* National Academy Press, Washington, D.C.
————. 1987b. *Improving research through peer review.* National Academy Press, Washington, D.C.

Crops, Congress, Consumers, Constituents: Some Comments on Context

M.M. Simpson

U.S. Congressional Research Service, CRS SPR LM413
Washington, D.C. 20540

Advances in the sciences today often occur not just in the laboratory but within an important social and political context. The transformation of agriculturally important crops is occurring not just in research settings but also in Congress, the regulatory agencies, and the world of the general public, domestically and internationally. Because regulatory issues are covered by other chapters in this volume, this paper briefly presents a perspective on transforming agriculturally important crops within the context of some currently important issues.

SUMMARY

This paper is the viewpoint of a specialist in life sciences in the U.S. Congressional Research Service (CRS). All members and committees of Congress can request information and analysis from CRS on all issues of interest to them. This information and analysis must be accurate, timely, objective, and balanced. It is from this perspective that the following comments on the context of transforming agriculturally important crops arose.

Six general and important context-setting issues are described: national and individual economic well-being and security, competitiveness, environmental protection, exogenous control, ethics in business, and concern about the irrational public. The transformation of agriculturally important crops is discussed briefly within the context of those six issues.

PERSPECTIVE

The perspective of this paper is from that of a specialist in life sciences in the U.S. Congressional Research Service (CRS), a part of the Library of Congress. The nearly 800 workers of CRS take as their principal mission to provide Congress with information and analysis on all issues of legislative interest. As part of that objective, this paper contains my views and opinions, which are not necessarily those of CRS or of the Congress.

CRS provides its assistance to Congress in several different ways, depending on time constraints, the wishes of the congressional client, and individual judgments as to the most effective method. We can provide assistance via written memoranda, short overviews called issue briefs, and compilations of information and analysis in "info packs." Analysis and information can be provided on audiotape and/or videotape for briefings via car tape players or office video recorders. Briefings can also be given over the telephone or in person. Assistance can be provided for hearings and for creating legislation.

All the work of CRS is in support of the legislative branch. It should be remembered that Congress creates laws and is one of our three major branches of government: The executive branch, which executes the laws, with assistance of the various agencies; the judicial branch, which interprets the laws; and the legislative branch.

At this time, Congress has no professional butchers, and no member made a living by baking. Of the 435 representatives and 100 senators, 246 termed their previous occupation "attorney." All are aware of the pressures of being an elected official and are beholden to divergent interests and interest groups. The purpose of this section is to illuminate my perspective and to begin to provide a context (that of the legislative branch of the federal government) within which to discuss the issue of the transformation of agriculturally important crops.

SIX CONTEXT-SETTING ISSUES
I have chosen six general and important context-setting issues: (1) national and individual economic well-being and security; (2) competitiveness; (3) environmental protection; (4) exogenous control; (5) ethics in business; and (6) concern about the irrational public.

National and Individual Economic Well-being and Security
Despite all rhetoric and actions to date, the federal deficit continues to grow. At the same time, the national trade deficit continues to be a problem, rising from $36 billion in 1980 to

$170 billion in 1986. Those and other concerns have added to the recent bumpiness of the stock market roller coaster. Our nation has a continuing problem with the homeless; the news undoubtedly again will carry stories of homeless individuals freezing to death in the coming winter. Finally, there has been no clear sign of a decrease in the dependence on welfare of the poor.

Within this economic context is the continuing issue of what to do about our agricultural sector. The record $26 billion in farm commodity programs was provided in 1986, amid low commodity prices, declining export sales, and increasing surpluses. Those working to transform agriculturally important crops should remember this economic context.

Competitiveness
The economic context provides a portion of this issue. But beyond the previous considerations, there is concern over the increasing number of foreign students in our institutions of higher learning, some of whom are paid to learn our most advanced knowledge to bring back to their homes for application. Consider the difficulty in retaining good researchers in academe, the argument that a variety of environmental and other regulations may be driving some research and production opportunities abroad and finally, certain import advantages and export restrictions that work to decrease domestic vitality.

Other considerations are the role of intellectual property protection and its effects on competitiveness, controls on imported commodities, the easing of certain export restrictions to increase export opportunities, and efforts to allow increased vertical integration in industries to enhance efficiency. These issues can be of vital importance to the transformation of important crops.

Environmental Protection
Over the years, we have evolved from concern about conventional pollutants, such as carbon monoxide and nitrogen oxides, to toxics, with chemical names abbreviated to a few letters, often to facilitate media coverage. There also has been evolution from concern about relatively local pollution effects, such as killer smogs in London and Donora, to transboundary pollution, such as international acid deposition, toxic pesticide residues, and transboundary pesticide pollution. Work in

transforming crops must be considered in light of these evolving concerns.

Exogenous Control
Much political and general attention has been focused on secret arms dealings with Iran. Now, with a retiring President, some cynics and others worry that the pressure may be irresistible to develop a secret arms treaty to ensure a noble place in history. Secret deals of this sort speak of a distrust and suspicion of exogenous control, of strings being pulled out of sight with uncontrollable outcomes.

Although allowing increased vertical integration in industries may enhance efficiency, there is concern that such integration may overly centralize agricultural economic power, a situation wherein secret deals and exogenous control may occur. There is concern that such integration may lead to a reduction in innovation. Transforming agricultural crops is one activity that may be involved in efforts to develop a new antitrust policy, one that prevents harm while increasing the benefits of big business.

Ethics in Business
Concerns about stockbrokers, corporate raiders, chief executive officers, and other powerful figures facing sanctions for illegal or unethical activities are the elements of this context-setting issue.

There are parallel concerns about the ethics of tinkering with the genes of plants, animals, or humans, perhaps epitomized by concerns about who should have ownership of genetic information. The concerns may be greatest for human genetic information, but similar consideration applies to plants as well.

Concern about the Irrational Public
Nuclear power and hazardous waste, symbolized by the incidents surrounding Three Mile Island and Love Canal, are just two examples of this issue, that of the public's acting and/or reacting from emotion and not rationality. Nuclear power and hazardous wastes exemplify the difficulties of dealing with the public on issues that may exist beyond reason and facts.

Relevant here are obvious concerns about deliberately releasing genetically engineered organisms. But beyond deliberate release, attention should be given to the power of advertising and media in general. Those working at transforming crops should be aware of the perceptions of the public and the shapers of those perceptions.

CONCLUSION
We do not live in a fairy-tale land with a benevolent monarch guiding us. We live in a complex and dynamic, democratically based society (one of many societies in the world) that moves in several directions, often at the same time, driven by myriad interests. This paper has attempted to describe briefly some contexts that may be important to the work of transforming agriculturally important crops.

Productivity Implications of Biotechnology

V.W. Ruttan

Department of Agricultural and Applied Economics
University of Minnesota, St. Paul
Minnesota 55108

In this paper, I cast the implications of current research in biotechnology for technical change and productivity growth in agriculture within a historical and global context. I then discuss some of my concerns about the potential for continued productivity growth in the U.S. agriculture.

The Rate and Direction of Agricultural Productivity Growth

Prior to the beginning of this century, almost all increases in agricultural production occurred as a result of increases in area cultivated. The major exceptions were in Western Europe, where livestock-based conservation systems of farming had developed, and in East Asia, where wet rice cultivation systems had developed. By the end of this century, there will be few significant areas where agricultural production can be expanded by simply adding more land to production. Expansion of agricultural output will have to be obtained almost entirely from more intensive cultivation of the areas already being used for agricultural production. Increases in food and fiber production will depend in large measure on continuous advances in agricultural technology.

At the risk of some oversimplification, it is useful to distinguish between advances in mechanical technology, which generate increases in output per worker, and advances in biological technology, which generate increases in output per hectare (Fig. 1). Figure 1 depicts the long-run patterns of growth in output per hectare and output per worker for Japan, Denmark, France, the United Kingdom, and the United States between 1880 and 1980. It also identifies the current levels of both output per worker and output per hectare for a number of other developed and developing countries. The story that emerges from Figure 1 is that almost from the beginning, Japan directed its technical development toward increasing

107

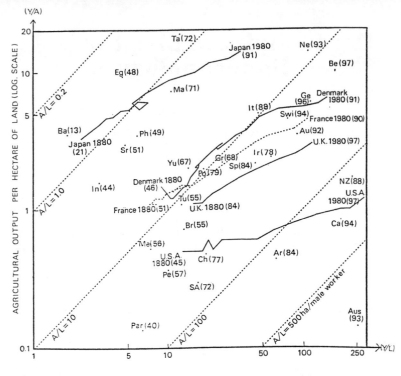

Figure 1 Historical growth paths of agricultural productivity of Denmark, France, Japan, the United Kingdom, and the United States for 1880–1980, compared with intercountry cross-section observations of selected countries in 1980. Values in parentheses are percentage of male workers employed in nonagriculture. (Reprinted, with permission, from Hayami and Ruttan 1985.)

Symbol Key: (Ar) Argentina; (Aus) Australia; (Au) Austria; (Ba) Bangladesh; (Be) Belgium (& Luxembourg); (Br) Brazil; (Ca) Canada; (Ch) Chile; (Co) Colombia; (De) Denmark; (Eg) Egypt; (Fi) Finland; (Fr) France; (Ge) Germany, F.R.; (Gr) Greece; (In) India; (Ir) Ireland; (Is) Israel; (It) Italy; (Ja) Japan; (Li) Libya; (Ma) Mauritius; (Me) Mexico; (Ne) Netherlands; (NZ) New Zealand; (No) Norway; (Pak) Pakistan; (Par) Paraguay; (Pe) Peru; (Ph) Philippines; (Po) Portugal; (SA) South Africa; (Sp) Spain; (Sr) Sri Lanka; (Su) Surinum; (Swe) Sweden; (Swi) Switzerland; (Sy) Syria; (Ta) Taiwan; (Tu) Turkey; (UK) U.K.; (USA) U.S.A.; (Ve) Venezuela; (Yu) Yugoslavia.

output per hectare. In contrast, the United States directed its efforts primarily to expanding output per worker (Ruttan 1981). Over the last several decades, the patterns of Japan and the United States have begun to converge.

Output per hectare and output per worker indicate the direction of technical change. They are both partial productivity measures. Efficiency is measured more appropriately in terms of changes in output per unit of total input. Average rates of change in output per unit of total input for U.S. agriculture for the period 1870–1980 are presented in Table 1. Prior to 1925, output per total unit of total input was primarily accounted for by advances in labor productivity. Since the mid-1920s, advances in land productivity have made an increasing contribution in growth in output. Note the very slow growth in productivity during the 1900–1925 period—between the closing of the frontier and the introduction of hybrid corn. Note the decline in the annual total productivity growth rates between the 1950–1965 period and the 1965–1982 period. Since the mid-1920s, advances in science-based technology have contributed to the transition of U.S. agriculture from a resource- to a science-based industry. This transition has only begun and has occurred at a somewhat slower pace in Western Europe and Japan. It has only begun in many parts of the developing world. Figure 1 shows that low levels of output per worker and per hectare occur in most developing countries. It is imperative over the next several decades that we complete the establish-

Table 1 Average Annual Rates of Change (Percentage per Year) in Output, Input, and Productivity in U.S. Agriculture, 1870–1982

Item	1870–1900	1900–1925	1925–1950	1950–1965	1965–1982
Farm output	2.9	0.9	1.6	1.7	2.1
Total input	1.9	1.1	0.2	-0.4	0.2
Total productivity	1.0	-0.2	1.3	2.2	1.8
Labor input[a]	1.6	0.5	-1.7	-4.8	-3.4
Labor productivity	1.3	0.4	3.3	6.6	5.8
Land input[b]	3.1	0.8	0.1	-0.9	0.0
Land productivity	-0.2	0.0	1.4	2.6	1.8

Sources: U.S. Department of Agriculture, *Economic Indicators of the Farm Sector: Production and Efficiency Statistics, 1980* (Washington, D.C.: U.S. Department of Agriculture, Economic Research Service, January 1982, and subsequent issues); U.S. Department of Agriculture, *Changes in Farm Production and Efficiency* (Washington, D.C.: 1979); and D.D. Durost and G.T. Barton, *Changing Sources of Farm Output* (Washington, D.C.: U.S. Department of Agriculture Production Research Report No. 36, February 1960). Data are 3-year averages centered on the year shown for 1925, 1950, and 1965.
[a]Number of workers, 1870–1910; worker-hour basis, 1910–1971.
[b]Cropland use for crops, including crop failures and cultivated summer fallow.

ment of agricultural research capacity for each commodity of economic significance in each agroclimatic region of the world (Ruttan 1986). A country that fails to evolve and sustain the capacity for technical and institutional innovation in agriculture consistent with its resource and cultural endowments will be unable to provide its farmers with the technology needed to meet the expectations that society will place on its agricultural sector.

Some Concerns about Productivity

The ability of the U.S. agricultural sector to sustain a rate of growth in total productivity, in output per unit of total input, that approaches the rate that has prevailed during the first three decades since World War II.

As a result of advances in biological technology associated with the new knowledge in molecular biology and its biotechnological applications, there has been a great deal of speculation to the effect that American agriculture may be confronted with a new burst of productivity growth that exceeds the rate of growth in demand for agricultural commodities. It is anticipated that advances in animal health and productivity will come first, followed by advances in plant protection and somewhat later by advances in plant productivity. But I see nothing in the evidence presented in this volume or in the recent rash of technology assessment studies that leads me to anticipate productivity gains over the next several decades comparable to the gains achieved since 1940 as a result of (1) the reduction in farm labor and work-animal input associated with mechanical technology and (2) the advances in crop yields and animal-feeding efficiency resulting from advances in plant and animal breeding and in crop and animal nutrition.

We can expect a slowing of additional gains from advances in mechanical technology. The cost of saving an additional man-day by adding more horsepower per worker has largely played itself out in countries like the United States, Canada, and Australia. I also have serious concerns about the rate of growth in output per hectare. Increases in crop yields during the last century of experimental breeding have been achieved primarily due to selection for a higher harvest index—by redistributing the dry matter between the vegetative and reproductive parts of the plant (Jain 1986). The harvest index has risen from the 20–30% range to upward of 50% for several major grain crops. There is growing concern that a plateau is

110

now being reached in yield potential based on failure, under experimental conditions, to push the harvest index much above 50%. If this is correct, it means that future gains in those countries that are currently pushing against the technological frontier will have to come from increases in total dry matter production from enhanced photosynthetic capacity.

The apparent inability to design a rational farm policy regime that can take effective advantage of our natural and scientific resource base.

In the mid-1970s, conferences devoted to the issues that we are discussing today were dominated by a pervasive pessimism regarding the adequacy of natural resource endowments and the supply of resource commodities and services. By the mid-1980s, the fear of scarcity had been replaced by a fear of abundance. This fear of abundance, in turn, has triggered a growth in agricultural protectionism in developed countries and has encouraged the development of increasingly expensive agricultural commodity programs in the United States, Western Europe, and Japan.

Two basic principles should guide the reform of agricultural commodity policy. The first is that we should move toward a policy environment in which agricultural commodities move across national borders at least as freely as financial resources. The second is that there should be a delinking of policies designed to provide income protection for farm families from policies designed to stabilize farm agricultural commodity markets.

Despite the jumble of target prices, loan rates, and deficiency payments, the basic mechanism used to achieve agricultural commodity price-policy objectives for the major field crops—wheat, corn, cotton, and rice—is renting land from farmers. The "rent" that induces a farmer to idle enough land to participate in a commodity program is referred to as "a deficiency payment." It is calculated as the difference between "a target price" and the loan rate multiplied by the normal yield on the eligible portion of the farmer's historical "base acreage." There is no way that a program that attempts to limit supply or enhance prices by renting land from farmers or by direct purchases of farm commodities can avoid incurring excessively high costs. And there is no way that such a program can avoid directing its benefits to the largest farmers. Most of the land or the commodities must be obtained from the

15–20% of all farmers, who account for 60–80% of production.

A first step that should be taken in any program designed to make more effective use of the resources and technology available to American farmers is to eliminate the price support loan rates. Elimination of the loan rates would permit dismantling the obsolete system of acreage allotments and "bases" on which the loans are based. It would permit production to shift to those areas where costs are lowest. It would permit agricultural commodities to move into international trade at market prices. The United States would no longer be forced to occupy the role of a residual supplier in world markets or to hold a price umbrella over producers in other countries.

Income support payments to farmers should be based on the difference between the market price and a "target price." The target price might initially be set at a level that would cover production costs on an efficient family farm. The price should be computed using a formula that would reflect both productivity growth and inflation rates. The payments should be subject to a limitation that reflects a much greater sense of equity among farm and nonfarm recipients of transfers of payment than the present $50,000 per farm limitation, which presently leaks at "at the top."

REFERENCES

Hayami, Y. and V. Ruttan. 1985. *Agricultural development: An international perspective.* John Hopkins University Press, Baltimore.

Jain, H.K. 1986. Eighty years of post-Mendelian breeding for crop yield: Nature of selection pressures and future potential. *Indian J. Genet. Plant Breed.* (suppl.) **46:** 30.

Ruttan, V.W. 1981. *Agricultural research policy, Minneapolis,* p. 17. University of Minnesota Press, St. Paul.

———. 1986. Toward a global agricultural research system: A personal view. *Res. Policy* **15:** 307.

Scientific, Economic, and Product Development Issues for Agronomic Crops

R.T. Fraley,[1] V.W. Ruttan,[2] N. Fedoroff,[3] and M. Simpson[4]

[1]Monsanto Company, St. Louis, Missouri 63198
[2]Department of Agricultural and Applied Economics, University of Minnesota, St. Paul, Minnesota 55108
[3]Department of Embryology, Carnegie Institution of Washington Baltimore, Maryland 21210
[4]United States Congressional Research Service Washington, DC 20540

The successful development and commercialization of genetically engineered plants represents a key issue for ensuring the future productivity of U.S. agriculture. A number of recent government and private reports have strongly advocated investment in agricultural biotechnology research to help meet growing competition for international and domestic markets from countries with developing production capabilities, cheaper labor pools, and/or strict trade policies. Many foresee the impact of biotechnology on agriculture to be as significant as farm mechanization, the development of hybrid crops, and the use of agrichemicals.

Ironically, it has been difficult to develop the strong, unified, pro-agricultural technology position in the U.S. necessary to expand technology development because of controversy and debate surrounding various social, political, and scientific policy issues. In the midst of current grain surpluses and concerns over the environmental aspects of certain agricultural technologies and the changing farm infrastructure, commitment to a long-term strategic vision for agricultural research and development is missing. Without such a commitment, the effort necessary to overcome technical, regulatory, commercial, and public acceptance hurdles may delay and diminish the beneficial impact of important new agricultural technologies. This is reflected in the fact that despite the enormous scientific advances made in the plant field during the last 5 years, federal support for basic agricultural research has not been significantly increased. Also, in just the last year, several major U.S. companies have decided to eliminate or divest themselves of their agricultural biotechnology programs. Meanwhile, nationally focused efforts have been initiated in Japan, China, and several European countries to develop and exploit these new technologies. These observations indicate the very fragile situation that currently exists and raise the question whether the window for the U.S. opportunity in agricultural biotechnology is beginning to close.

Rather than debating the validity or cause of these various complicated issues, the panel addressed specific areas that should be considered as initiatives to improve this situation. The intent is to develop a balanced, but advocative environment to ensure that potential regulatory, commercial, and public acceptance hurdles do not delay and diminish the beneficial impact of agricultural biotechnology.

National Emphasis on Agricultural Research and Development

Currently, U.S. agriculture has a tarnished image and only fragmented political and commercial support. The focus on short-term issues is obscuring the need for continued science and technology development to ensure that an abundant, safe, nutritious, high-quality, and low-cost food supply is maintained. Negative aspects (grain surpluses, ground-water contamination, release of genetically engineered organisms, loss of family farms, price supports, antitechnology sentiments, etc.) have almost completely overshadowed the positive aspects of new agricultural technologies (more competitive U.S. agricultural production systems, lower food costs, ability to meet worldwide food demand, more jobs, enhanced environmental acceptability, etc.). Preservation of our food supply and agricultural competitiveness needs to be studied at the highest levels of government and policy making.

Possible Actions. Individual scientists, professional societies, companies, and industrial associations should persuade government agencies and key political figures to position "preservation of the food supply and U.S. agricultural competitiveness" as a priority issue. Analyses should be carried out to evaluate thoroughly the positive impact of agricultural biotechnology on issues such as employment, natural resource conservation, and long-term competitiveness in international markets; this information should be made widely available.

Involvement of the Agricultural Scientific Community in Education and Policy Making

Several of the discussions showed the failure of agricultural scientists and their professional societies to take an aggressive lead role in public education and policy-making activities. Sometimes not a single response was received to notices in the *Federal Register* outlining proposed new regulations that have significantly affected agricultural research. Many other professional disciplines have monitoring and lobbying functions to ensure that careful attention is focused on such issues. The complexity of today's regulatory environment and the vulnerability of individual scientists or research programs to political and social events warrant a careful reexamination of the role of professional societies in this capacity.

Possible Actions. The agricultural scientific community should identify and appropriately staff offices within professional societies or industrial associations to monitor proposed guidelines and new regulations and to disseminate information and recommendations to its members. This function should serve as the focal point both for organizing responses to proposed regulations and petitions to modify inappropriate policies and for informing members of important changes in the regulatory process.

Increased Awareness of Unique Aspects of Agricultural Research by Regulatory Agencies

The general consensus of the meeting participants was that the agencies (USDA, EPA, and FDA) involved in regulation of agricultural biotechnology products have made considerable progress in defining their respective organizational structures and in providing a basic framework for release of genetically modified plants. Three issues discussed were felt to be particularly important areas for continued advancement.

The *first* issue was to recognize the need for defining a progression of regulatory requirements ranging from small-scale field testing to product development and commercial scale. It was generally believed that the risks associated with release of genetically engineered plants in the environment was quite low and that small-scale field experiments in particular posed little cause for concern and should require minimal regulatory oversight. The petition process of the USDA represents one approach to reducing unnecessary or modifying inappropriate regulations. The view was expressed that it would be appropriate for the various agencies to institute an internal process to review and examine regulations periodically as more experience and knowledge is gained from research and from the field testing of genetically engineered plants.

The *second* issue dealt with the need for individual agencies to formulate specific guidelines and regulations dealing with the commercialization of genetically engineered plants. A concern was expressed that the technology is developing faster than expected and that issues such as regulatory costs, testing requirements, and timelines are now becoming important factors in the decision to commercialize genetically engineered plants. In formulating their requirements, the agencies must recognize both the inherent low risk of this technology and the fact that the seed industry simply cannot support a regulatory framework similar to that of the drug and agrichemical industries.

A *third* issue was that of making all parties aware of the need to develop a regulatory framework for commercializing genetically engineered plants without drawing unnecessary attention to the particular biotechnology process used to improve crop plants. The point was raised that simply labeling a genetically engineered plant as containing a food additive or being different from current crops in any way would probably be sufficient to deter acceptance in the marketplace.

Possible Actions. Conferences similar to this one which bring together scientific, regulatory, and commercial representatives are an excellent means to communicate issues and information. Although there have been several conferences on subjects relating to intentional release of genetically engineered organisms and risk assessment, there are very few meetings that target the beneficial impact of the technology. It is recommended that Cold Spring Harbor/Banbury Center initiate an annual meeting to focus on subjects promoting the development, commercialization, and consumer acceptance of agricultural biotechnology products.